LOGIC, MIND & HEALTH

Moving Beyond Stress to a Happier, More Purposeful Life

Brandon Hall

© 2019, Brandon Hall

ISBN (paperback): 978-0-578-57790-6

ISBN (eBook): 978-0-578-60639-2

Library of Congress Control Number: 2019918882

Cover and design by Mike Bohrer, Debra Hall and Dan Orloff

For more information, visit www.logicmindandhealth.com

Printed in the United States of America

Kulpsville, Pennsylvania

Contents

Thinking

Daily Routine

An Argument for the Existence and Nature of God

Free Will and Leibniz Optimism

Craig's Philosophy

Hope, Thought, and Belief

Acknowledgments

This book, along with everything else I do in life, is dedicated to my family—my ultimate purpose.

To my editor, Pamela Feinsilber—you are simply awesome. Thank you for sorting through the barrage of information in my brain and helping me bring this book to life.

A special thanks to all my friends from the Mentee Inner Circle for the guidance, support, and encouragement. You helped make it possible for me to take action and pursue my passion.

To those of you who are suffering from stress or hardship—I feel you. To those who may be skeptical about your ability to improve your life, or fear change, or are reluctant to reach out for help—please do try. You can change your brain, your habits, your relationships with the people around you, and live a better, more fulfilled life.

And, thank you, God.

Forward

In my career as a cardiac-device specialist, I have seen thousands of people who wouldn't be alive today without their pacemakers or defibrillators. They have literally been given another chance at life, and they know it. Many have expressed regret to me about the unhealthy way they treated their bodies.

That's why it's hard for me to see people try to manage their stress by using unhealthy, counterproductive coping mechanisms, like overindulging in junk food and sweets, or self-medicating with alcohol or drugs. Clearly, there are better, more effective ways to deal with stress. Often, as in my case, the stress is self-inflicted and comes from a fearful mindset. This is one of the many reasons I decided to write a book sharing what I have learned about chronic stress, how to manage it, and, in fact, how to live a better life.

I've witnessed the traumatic effect that stress can have on the human body. Each of my parents, who had always been in good physical health, was diagnosed with cancer at age 50, immediately following major stressful events in their lives. I have no doubt that unmitigated stress was one of the main triggers, if not the main trigger, for this ugly illness.

My mom has carried stress with her from as far back as her childhood. She came from a home plagued with substance abuse, physical and verbal abuse, anger, and eventually a divorce that separated her and her siblings. While she overcame those beginnings to create a beautiful family of her own, they shaped a high-strung personality. Issues big and small became instant stressors, particularly if they involved her husband or children.

My dad's stress developed from the day-to-day weight of taking care of his wife and kids and dealing with challenging work environments. Bit by bit, the unchecked stresses of everyday life accumulated, compounded, and ultimately wore him down.

My parents' stress probably shaped some of my own stress and fear, although I certainly don't fault them for it, because I know it wasn't intentional. They absolutely showered my siblings and me with love. But the stress was always there, and we never really knew how to deal with it.

Watching your parents battle cancer is a terrible experience. Thankfully, after various treatments, they are both alive and well. But after seeing what they went through, I felt compelled to better understand how to take control of and mitigate stress. I wanted to help others—and myself—become more aware of stressful mindsets before they affect our precious health and well-being.

The first section of this book looks at how the brain works, its influence on our conscious and unconscious emotions and behavior, its malleability or neuroplasticity, and how we can change an unhealthy, habitual mindset. I came to feel that it's not enough to manage our stress, however; that to truly overcome our self-inflicted chronic stress, we need to change the way we think about the world. The second section looks at notions of happiness, the importance of meaning and purpose in one's life, and what I call living a transcendent life.

I've labeled the first section Physiology and the second one Philosophy, and both are bolstered with scientific research—for instance, one recent study has shown that having a sense of life purpose has a greater effect on longevity than regular exercise or even not smoking.

The third section details the stress-reducing practices I use, from deep breathing, visualization, and progressive muscle relaxation to my "keystone habits," meditation and mindfulness. These, too, are validated by scientific research.

None of this information should be taken as medical advice. I believe in talking to a professional about any physical, mental, or emotional challenges you may be trying to deal with. Please consult your physician before you commence any new health-related activities.

I am not a doctor, a scientist, a philosopher, or a psychologist. I am just a guy who grew up around and suffered from fear and stress for a long time. I had to do something about it, because of the toll it was taking on my health, my work, and my family life. I can't help but think of the biblical notion "to whom much is given, much is expected." I have been beyond blessed in my life, and now it is my turn to give in a greater capacity than I ever have.

Prologue

Fear has plagued most of my adult life, dating back to college. I was fortunate enough to play Division I football at an academically rigorous school. This opportunity was an absolute blessing, but I found the pressure of succeeding on the field and in the classroom overwhelming. I was afraid of letting the people in my life down, which led to hesitation on the field and poor grades in the classroom. I wouldn't ask for help or ask questions for fear of appearing dumb in front of my peers. I was afraid to disappoint my coaches, so I said yes to whatever they asked me to do, which included playing different positions, even when I didn't enjoy them.

I was so stressed out on the nights before tests, I couldn't remember any of the material I was trying to learn. So nervous during practice and before games, I forgot the plays. So worried that I would make a mistake, I prayed the game would end before I even got in to play. I wished many of my most precious college moments away because I was too afraid to face them.

Nobody taught me how to deal with my lack of confidence, manage my stress, and enjoy the incredible opportunity I had at that time in my life. I could have created better outcomes on the field and in the classroom had I been able to communicate effectively with my coaches and professors. My challenge was not the people in my life or the situations I faced, but rather my own internal-processing system. My stress was entirely self-inflicted. It came from my own fearful ways of thinking.

I carried that fear into the corporate world and to an extremely challenging job. For over 10 years, I worked as a certified cardiac-device specialist, serving in a clinical sales role for a company that provides pacemakers and implantable defibrillators to patients with various heart-related illnesses. The job put me in the operating room, running the medical equipment. That hands-on part of the job was remarkably fulfilling, yet extremely stressful. During the procedure, if a patient was dependent on the medical device to keep their heart beating (which was often the case), I literally held their life in the palm of my hand.

Another aspect of the procedure involved a requirement to test the equipment to make sure it was not defective. That involved pressing a button to effectively kill the person (put them into ventricular fibrillation, a life-ending heart arrhythmia if left untreated) until the device brought them back to life with a shock. If you have ever seen medical personnel on TV, with their hand-held pads placed on someone's chest and yelling "Clear!" as they try to shock the patient back to life, that is essentially what the little implantable defibrillators do. And I was the one initiating the shock. As you might imagine, there is a little bit of stress involved with that procedure, too!

In many instances, the patients were in hospice care and we were required to turn off their defibrillation therapy. This is routine, to ensure the device will not intervene to save them when their heart begins to fail. This usually involved being in a room with family members staring at you as if you were the Grim Reaper. Even though the deactivation doesn't cause the patient's death, it was one of the toughest things I ever had to do. The emotion in the room was enough to make me cry, too. And sometimes I did.

I thoroughly enjoyed many aspects of the job, like the patient interactions and helping to save lives. But over the years, the chronic stress and fear took its toll. My blood pressure shot through the roof; I had trouble focusing and remembering things; it was hard to relax. To alleviate the stress, I turned to physical coping mechanisms, mainly sugar. My favorite way to cope was with Oreo cookies, and lots of them, Double Stuffed preferred. I could easily open a package and inhale a row or two in three minutes flat.

My wife could always tell when I had had a bad day, because she'd catch me standing in the pantry when I should've been playing with the kids or helping around the house. "Whatcha doin' in there?" she'd ask in a joking manner. Slamming cookies, of course. I'd poke my head out the door, frown, and stick it right back into the package.

The cookies brought me great pleasure in the short term, but of course they did more harm than good. I often had night sweats from overeating, and I soon carried several extra pounds, especially around my midsection.

When I couldn't stand to look at myself in the mirror with my shirt off, I went the opposite route. I had smoothies for breakfast and ate mostly salads and vegetables, with a bit of lean meat, for lunch and dinner. I started going to the gym several times a week and lifting heavy weights again, like in football. That worked much better than the sugar to calm my nerves, but the fear remained, the stress always came back, and the vicious circle continued.

One of the benefits of my job was years of education about anatomy, physiology, and heart-healthy actions, like diet and exercise. I started talking to people I associated with—particularly the physicians I saw on a daily basis. I asked them about chronic stress, the true nature of lifestyle-related illness, and health-improvement practices beyond diet and exercise. They introduced me to Western and Eastern medical practices, natural healing remedies, and philosophical thought, which really piqued my interest.

In the end, if I had to choose one word for what I learned, it is *self-awareness*. I realized that I was just trying to get by, trying to bury the fear and put on a happy face, not living my life to its fullest. I needed to find a real, long-term solution.

Part 1: Physiology - Stress and the Brain

The Three Brains

Everything in our lives begins and ends in the brain. Its main task is to keep us alive and safe. It is the reason we jump out of the way when a car is speeding toward us, the reason we don't grab that hot pan without wearing oven mitts. Unfortunately, because it locks in thoughts and actions that aren't as helpful as these, the brain is also at the center of our habitual stress and anxiety.

I found this out in my first year as a certified cardiac-device specialist. I worked in a clinical sales role for a company that provides pacemakers and implantable defibrillators to patients with heart-related illnesses. Part of the job entailed running medical equipment in the operating room—literally controlling a person's heartbeat.

During the pacemaker-implant procedure, the physician places wires directly into a patient's heart through a vein up near the shoulder. In this particular case, the patient's heart was in an extremely vulnerable state. The slightest disturbance by a wire in a certain area of the heart could result in a flatline (no heartbeat). And that's exactly what happened. And no one saw it but me.

These are such routine procedures, and cardiologists are quite used to that type of heart condition. That day, everyone was talking, working, not really paying attention to the EKG monitor displaying the patient's heart rhythm. But somehow, as the physician was manipulating the wire, the patient's heart stopped. Just like you see in movies and shows on TV, the flat green line ran across the screen.

A rush of adrenaline hit me immediately. I could feel my chest tighten, my heart rate increase—it was as if I was the one having heart trouble! I knew exactly what I was supposed to do, but I froze. My brain froze, too. Even though I had received extensive training for that exact situation, I had no idea what to do. I kept hoping someone else would say or do something, because I was the new guy. Who was I to speak up during a procedure?

After a few endless seconds, one of the nurses yelled, "Asystole!" (The medical term for flatlining.) There was a sudden silence, followed by an explosion of action and screaming. The screaming was mostly coming from the physician, yelling at me to do my job, which was to start the patient's heart back up. Yes, that was *my* job, because it was my equipment hooked up to the wire he placed in the patient's heart, the one that had caused the flatlining.

As soon as I heard the physician yelling, "Do your job!" I hit a little button on the equipment; this started the patient's heart beating again, and he was fine. But I certainly wasn't. Heart pounding, body sweating, I was shaking for the rest of the day. I carried that fearful experience with me to every single procedure, similar or not, for months. I thought about it every morning as I drove to work. I thought about it during the day and lying in bed at night. It was hard to relax because I was constantly on edge; even when I wasn't consciously thinking about what had occurred, I felt a sense of anxiety. Though the physician didn't reprimand me, and I never made that mistake again, I beat myself up over and over. And the more I relived that event, the more encoded it became in my brain and my body.

It was actually my brain's way of keeping me safe. As I learned later, there was a fascinating physiological reason why my brain held onto those emotions and stressful memories.

Because its main task is to keep us alive, the brain perceived that experience as a potential threat to survival. (Yes, *my* survival, not the patient's.) That's because if we vividly remember something that frightened us or caused us pain, it increases the likelihood that we will avoid it in the future. Think how easy it is to recall exactly where you were and what you were doing when a traumatic event occurred, whether the death of a loved one or a national emergency. With its cascade of powerful thoughts and emotions, that event encoded a strong memory within your brain.[1]

For the sake of simplicity, we'll consider three general regions of the brain involved in this process of memory formation, conscious thought, emotion, and behavior: the cortex (let's call it the logical brain), the limbic system (the emotional brain), and the brain stem (the primal brain). They evolved separately over eons of time.[2]

The oldest region, the primal brain, is located just above the spinal cord, toward the back of the head. It is vital for basic biological mechanisms that promote survival, such as heart rate, respiratory rate, temperature, and balance. It runs automatically, so we don't have to consciously think about breathing or remind our hearts to beat.

Just above the primal brain, the emotional brain plays an integral role in the way we behave, react, and remember things. It is where we feel love and hate, anger and fear, joy and sorrow. As neuroscientist Selena Bartlett, PhD, puts it in her helpful book

Smashing Mindset: Train Your Brain to Reboot, Recharge, Reinvent Your Life, "It's also where we make judgments about ourselves and the world: When we decide whether something is safe to eat or a stranger is friend or foe, we are using this part of the brain."[3]

An important part of the limbic or emotional brain is the amygdala. This is a region of the brain that helps encode those powerful memories, and it is extremely active during stressful situations. We remember some experiences as vividly as we do because in order to survive, our ancestors had to remember their moments of fear and danger. It would be of no benefit to the survival of our species if, after hunting, our ancient ancestors forgot about being chased by a saber-tooth tiger. Or if, when they were scavenging for food and accidentally ate some poisonous berries, they did not notice which berries were harmful. They would certainly want to remember these experiences on their next excursions into the wild.

The cortex, or logical brain, is the outer layer of the brain. The other two, older regions tend to work unconsciously, but the cortex is the seat of our conscious thinking and awareness. It is involved in impulse control, emotional management, rationality, and planning. While it works more slowly than the other regions, it oversees them and helps them work together. But only if we let it.

Conscious vs. Unconscious Brain Function

Neuroscience research has established that the vast majority of brain activity occurs below our conscious awareness.[4] And the brain's unconscious processing is about a million times more powerful than its conscious processing.[5] Just think about all the things that occurred in your environment while you were reading this—all of the sounds, smells, and other environmental stimuli your brain had to process without your knowing it. Think of all the biological functions your body performed without your having to think about them. Or the emotional state you find yourself in right now, which you didn't generate consciously.

So, the vast majority of the time, the parts of our brain associated with emotion are operating without our conscious awareness. Yes, we can consciously affect our emotions, but when we are not in tune with or aware of our internal states of being, our emotional brains are running the show. And if we are chronically stressed out, that is exactly what will continue to happen, unless, of course, we do something about it.

Because the emotional brain is fast and extremely powerful, it can override the logical brain. So often, we do things because we *feel* like it or because it *feels* good, not because we've used our better judgment (our logical brains). Think about impulse buying or indulging in a dessert after an already huge dinner. I think of all the Oreos I ate after that terrible day in the operating room. I knew that eating so many cookies was not good for my health or my waistline, but it sure did *feel* good.

My conscious, logical brain reminded me that I was well trained and that such an event was unlikely to ever happen again. But every time I walked into an operating room, even months later, my emotional brain triggered the fear and anxiety I felt. No matter how often I tried to tell myself how foolish that was, the emotions kept coming back. Then I would dwell on what had happened, making it even worse by reinforcing the negative emotions and perpetuating the fear. And then out came the cookies.

So: Our emotions drive much of our behavior, and the parts of the brain involving our emotions act mostly unconsciously. Pretty scary if you think about it. This is the challenge we face: If we don't take action to manage our emotional brains and reduce the stress in our lives, it becomes harder and harder to use our logical brains to keep our thoughts and emotions in check. It's a vicious cycle, actually, because the functioning of the logical brain is severely hampered by chronic stress.

The Stress Response
During an intense emotional experience, the parts of the brain below the cortex pump out stress hormones, such as cortisol, and neurotransmitters, like noradrenaline, causing the physical sensations that initiate the fight-or-flight response, also known as the stress response. Adrenaline and cortisol cause the release of glucose from our organs and tissues into the bloodstream. The glucose provides immediate energy for our muscles, so that we can get *moving*. For the same reason, heart and respiratory rates increase, heart contractions strengthen, our blood pressure goes up, and our muscles tense. In addition, our pupils dilate to enhance our vision, and extreme focus sets in. Other biological functions shut down or become greatly reduced in order to conserve energy for the upcoming encounter.[6]

The phrase has been updated to the fight-flight-freeze response, and the new word certainly indicates what I did in that operating room. In addition to preparing us for fight or flight, the stress response severely reduces our mental capability, because when danger is present, it is not a time for thinking. It is a time to react quickly and save oneself. Any thoughts that aren't geared toward protection are diminished, which is why it is so hard to learn and function normally in stressful situations.

The stress response is a brilliant mechanism for keeping us alive and safe, but when it's overused, it becomes the opposite: a major harm to our health. The sad part is, we often activate the stress response ourselves, with our own thoughts, emotions, and memories, over and over and over again. When we revisit an unhappy memory, such as abuse or divorce, or worry about a future occurrence, like a presentation or meeting at work, our emotions alone will trip the fight-or-flight mechanism and get those stress hormones pumping. And if cortisol is constantly present in high amounts in the bloodstream, it can lead to physical and emotional problems such as headaches, heart disease, anxiety, depression, and memory impairment.[7,8]

When the amygdala is overactive, it sends signals to the cortex to slow down or do less. In other words, chronic stress impairs the logical brain. When our ancestors were facing life-and-death situations on a daily basis, the emotional parts of the brain immediately and unconsciously generated the stress response to promote their survival. This was a good thing!

Today, though, we don't need to run from tigers; we rarely

have to dodge an oncoming car. Our stress more often comes from a difficult job, an unhappy marriage, rowdy kids we can't control. There's no good reason to dwell on a chewing out at work or a one-time mistake. That stress doesn't contribute to our survival—far from it. But our brains don't differentiate between hungry tigers and angry bosses. And the stress-response mechanism is as active in us as it was in our ancestors.

Brain Waves

The brain is composed of individual nerve cells, or neurons, that communicate through electrical charges by way of specialized connections called synapses. As it governs, initiates, and responds to all our biological functions, the brain is vibrating at specific frequencies, in states ranging from relaxation to high arousal, which our thoughts and emotions can affect. These vibrating frequencies, which are measured in hertz (Hz) using a machine called an electroencephalograph, or EEG, are known as brain-wave states.[9] From lowest frequency to high, the predominant types of brain-wave states are:

    * Delta (measured at 0.5 to 4 Hz): These are the slowest recorded brain waves; we're in this brain-wave state when asleep or unconscious.

    * Theta (4–8 Hz): We're in this frequency range when we're daydreaming or semiconscious; in this state, we're deeply and highly suggestible.

* Alpha (8–12 Hz): This frequency range is the bridge between our conscious and unconscious minds; with this range, we're still very relaxed, with just a little information being processed but much retained.

* Beta (12–30 Hz): In this frequency range, we're at our most focused, processing information, solving problems, completing tasks.

These are general descriptions, and reactions can vary with the frequency. For instance, using an EEG, one can observe higher beta ranges in someone during a stressful situation. Focus is generally heightened during the stress response, but after a while, such a high arousal state ceases to be useful for learning or problem solving. That brain-wave state requires a lot of energy to maintain and, with the help of the survival chemicals produced during the stress response, knocks the body out of balance.[10]

Most of the time I worked as a cardiac-device specialist, I knew that high-beta feeling all too well. I felt like my brain and body were running at high speed the entire day. Literally running—I can't tell you how many days I would sprint from one hospital to the next to cover a procedure, because I was afraid that if one of my colleagues was there instead, we would lose the next case to a competitor.

The business was extremely competitive. The sales reps working with other pacemaker companies had been on the job three to four times longer than I had, and they had very good relationships with all our customers. In sales, you get paid for the number of procedures you do, and typically, the physicians chose which rep they wanted to work with for each procedure.

That is why I *had* to be there in person, myself. After all, I was in sales, and it was my job to do the selling. That was best done by being in front of the customers and providing the best possible service for them and their patients. Doing implants was one of the best opportunities to do just that, which meant being in the operating room for every single pacemaker and defibrillator. It wasn't because my colleagues were unqualified to be in there. It was because I was afraid my customers would think I had something more important to do, and that it would cost my company business.

I made my workload overwhelming by trying to do it all. Even so, it wasn't the actual workload that was stressing me out, because I did have help. It wasn't pressure from my manager, because I had demonstrated success and was hitting our sales marks. (He was actually very supportive.) It wasn't my competition, because our company was doing well. It wasn't my customers, because they were fine having my colleagues cover the procedures. It was my own misperceptions causing me all that stress.

For years, I ran through walls to get the job done. And for years, I had a lot of success operating at this speed. But by the end of most days, my brain was in a fog; I could barely remember what I'd had for lunch that day. The high-beta-energy drain, combined with the emotional stress of the job—not to mention constantly reliving the heart-stopping incident, and others—left me craving sugar when I got home. And the Oreos were always happy to greet me.

Brain Waves and Suggestibility

Between birth and about two years of age, the human brain predominantly operates in delta waves. Between two and six years of age, the brain moves into the slightly higher theta-wave state.[11] Recall that theta brain-wave states are associated with high suggestibility and unconscious processing. That's why we say young children are like sponges: Without even trying, they're absorbing information from the external environment and the people they interact with—forming memories of experiences they will carry into adulthood, creating the foundations of their personalities and behavior.[12]

For those who have young kids, it is vitally important to understand that your every interaction with them is literally shaping their brains. Through your words and actions, you're affecting their psychological and social development, their minds and their futures.

I saw this clearly when I taught my son to wrestle—no, not as in World Wrestling Entertainment, but rather the roughhousing kind of play in the basement after work. I was a huge wrestling fan growing up, and some of my best memories are of wrestling around with my dad. I wanted to share that experience with my son. But after we'd been roughhousing for a few weeks, he began randomly giving me a nice welcome-home punch to the gut as soon as I walked in the door. He was and is a sweet, loving boy, but I had accidentally suppressed his kindness a bit and conditioned him to become a little bruiser.

He was about four years old, and I distinctly remember that he had never come after me in an aggressive manner before then. Wrestling and roughhousing had not been programmed into his behavior by anything other than me. Our family had never talked about wrestling; it was never on our TV; he'd shown zero interest in it until I started wrestling with him after work. Thankfully, my wife noticed the change and we were able to correct the behavior. And I started paying a lot more attention to my words and actions when I was around my kids.

Because their logical brains are not completely developed yet, children can't entirely understand the situations they face or what they hear from parents and others. (In fact, parts of the cortex are not fully developed until we reach our mid-twenties.[13]) That's why if we joke with our kids about the boogeyman, they will start sleeping with the light on! They don't have the thought-processing ability to tell us to stop messing with them until they are approaching the age of seven or so. Even adolescent brains are operating in a low brain-wave state (during which, remember, they are highly suggestible) and are not yet fully capable of rational understanding.[14]

More important, we often remain unaware of important, long-ago events and memories. Trauma that occurs during early childhood is essentially like a program downloaded onto the brain's hard drive. The unconscious memories of these adverse childhood experiences (ACE) not only can persist through adulthood, they can affect us physiologically, as well as emotionally.

Physical Effects of Stress

Every day, we face environmental stressors, such as toxins, mold, radiation, and weather conditions, that can affect our health and well-being. The chronic stress that burdens us, however, comes from our internal environment, in the form of upsetting thoughts, feelings, and emotions. Memories of traumatic childhood events are a particularly serious source of stress.

Pediatrician Nadine Burke Harris, M.D., has conducted extensive research on adverse childhood experiences and their effects, particularly on one's health and well-being later in life. In *The Deepest Well: Healing the Long-Term Effects of Childhood Adversity*, she describes how factors such as emotional and physical abuse, neglect, violence, and divorce can affect a child's physical development.

In one study, when children who had suffered adverse experiences or trauma were placed in an MRI, their brains showed measurable change. In particular, the hippocampus, a part of the limbic or emotional brain involved in learning and memory, was smaller than in the control group, whose members had no history of trauma. When these children had a second MRI done, 12 to 18 months later, it showed the hippocampus was even smaller. These findings suggest that the stress from the childhood trauma was still acting on the neurological system. Not surprisingly, the children with ACE had higher levels of cortisol (the "stress hormone") than the control group.

Similarly, recall the amygdala. This part of the emotional brain, which helps encode memories, is very active during stressful situations. MRI studies of children who had been maltreated in Romanian orphanages showed significant enlargement of the amygdala.[15]

The amygdala helps identify threats in the environment, but

when chronically activated due to stress, it begins incorrectly assessing what is threatening and what is not. It sends false alarms to other parts of the brain, highlighting things that should not be scary. That's why these children had chronic high levels of cortisol. If you are chronically stressed, about your job or anything else, you likely have a high level of cortisol, too.

As I mentioned earlier, the stress response releases noradrenaline, which also compromises the ability of the cortex to override emotional impulses triggered by the amygdala. For some people, that results in an inability to solve problems; with others, in aggressive and impulsive behavior. Either way, it is not helpful.

Stress hormones can also suppress immune function, leading to a weakened response to fighting everything from the common cold to tumors. Just as the brain has not fully developed in children, neither has the immune system—so when children are exposed to chronic stress, it can cause a lifelong alteration in their immune systems. Stress causes inflammation, and the greater amount of inflammation in the body, the greater the chance the body will attack itself. This can lead to autoimmune diseases.

Chronic stress can even affect our DNA. The strings of chromosomes that house our DNA are protected at each end by something called telomeres, which are like the plastic tips on a shoelace. Telomeres keep the chromosomes from deteriorating or running into the next-door chromosomes; they are the reason that each time a chromosome is replicated, the copy is true to the original.

You can probably guess what I'm going to say next: that the

biochemical effects of chronic stress are damaging to these end caps. If the caps, or telomeres, are too heavily damaged, they can shorten, and the cells can age prematurely or function in a way that leads to disease and even a shorter lifespan. Early childhood adversity is predictive of shorter telomeres later in life, again showing how detrimental childhood stress is on an adult's health and well-being.

Unhealthy Coping Mechanisms

Childhood traumas are not the only sources of stress, of course. The loss of a loved one, a debilitating injury, a painful or prolonged divorce, or, as in my case, a challenging job can encode powerful emotions and memories.

And many people are like I was, lacking self-awareness and unable to realize the effect the memories and resulting stress are having on us. Every time I thought about my experience in the operating room, when I froze instead of doing my job, I felt the same physical response: tight chest, shortness of breath, pounding heart, sweaty hands. Biochemically speaking, there was absolutely no reason for that. In her fascinating book *My Stroke of Insight: A Brain Scientist's Personal Journey*, neuroscientist Jill Bolte Taylor, PhD, concludes that the biochemical response to an emotion lasts about 90 seconds. After that, the body essentially dissipates the chemicals released, and the automatic emotional response is over.[16]

So, there's another reason stressful emotions seem to last so long: We allow ourselves to remain in an emotional state far longer than those 90 seconds. If it isn't bad enough that we unconsciously store the negative emotion in our brains, we often consciously replay that experience over and over again, retriggering the actual emotion. Instead of using our conscious brains to manage our emotional brains and working to prevent our stress, we perpetuate it.

Like many others, I sought to cope with my stress through something that brought me pleasure, namely sugar. When there weren't any Oreos left in the house, I'd grab whatever piece of chocolate or candy I could find. Dr. Bartlett explains why in *Smashing Mindset*: "Just as some parts of the brain respond to stress chemicals, like cortisol, others respond to pleasure or reward chemicals, such as dopamine. In an effort to keep itself alive, the brain balances the stress chemicals with feel-good chemicals."[17]

Sugar, alcohol, nicotine, and fatty, greasy foods all activate those "feel-good chemicals." For me, each bite of an Oreo, or a Kit-Kat bar or a gummy worm, was an influx of feel-good chemicals to counterbalance the stress chemicals.

And there's one more reason that I craved sugar. During the stress response, the body releases insulin, a hormone responsible for managing blood-sugar levels. Again, think of the body's fight-or-flight response: Stress frees the glucose for use in the muscles, so that we can run from danger. When the muscles don't use that glucose and the body does not expend that energy, the insulin drives it into the fat-storage cells—especially around the midsection—to be used later.[18]

Because the glucose is now stored in the fat cells, our blood sugar is low—another reason we tend to crave sweets when we're stressed out. High cortisol levels also cause the body to break down protein into glucose for energy use, as well as to move fat into the abdominal area as a reserve.[19]

It was pretty eye-opening when I learned about the biological mechanism that was fueling my sugar dominance. Not only were the cookies causing me to become fat, so was the stress that was driving me to eat them! The change in my blood sugar in response to the stress caused me to crave sweets, as did the surge of dopamine I received.

Though the brain tries to help us manage our stress, we wind up choosing unhealthy sources of relief. What we want to do is learn to preempt those negative, often unconscious thoughts and emotions that have us reaching for a cookie or a drink or blowing off steam by getting angry. What we want to do is use our logical brains—our conscious thinking—to stop those unhealthy automatic responses and create healthier habits. We want to change our brains!

Neuroplasticity, or Changing the Brain

Everyone understands the concept of changing your mind: You decide to order the steak instead of the chicken; you're getting ready to go out on a cold, rainy night until you opt to stay home and watch a movie. While it's a little more difficult, you can also *change your brain*—that is, with effort and practice, you can form new synapses, or neural connections, between the nervous system and the brain.

Remember the examples involving the hippocampus and the amygdala? And how the size of each of these brain structures has been shown to change under chronic stress? That is because the brain is malleable.

This changing or rewiring of the brain is referred to as neuroplasticity. Michael M. Merzenich, PhD, a neuroscientist and professor emeritus at the University of California, San Francisco, describes changes demonstrated by research on brain plasticity in his book *Soft-Wired: How the New Science of Brain Plasticity Can Change Your Life*. We know the brain's individual nerve cells, or neurons, communicate through electrical charges by way of the synapses.[20] Merzenich writes that we can strengthen the connections between neurons and enhance the brain areas that support learning and memory processes.[21]

How? There is a term in neuroscience known as Hebb's Law, which states that "nerve cells that fire together, wire together." In other words, the more a group of brain cells works together—like during the stress response—the easier it becomes to do so in the future. Neurons that have fired many times in the same ways organize into specific patterns with long-lasting connections.[22]

Repetition is key, and in some cases, repetitive thinking is all it takes to rewire the brain. Consider a 1995 study at the National Institute of Neurological Disorders and Stroke, National Institutes of Health, in Bethesda, Maryland. For five days, the subjects rehearsed piano exercises for two hours a day—in their minds. Brain scans showed physical changes in the areas responsible for those particular movements—the same brain changes as those who physically performed the same movements for the same period of time—even though they never lifted a finger![23]

These pianists were practicing the art of visualization, also referred to as mental imagery or mental rehearsal. Michael Phelps, the most decorated Olympian of all time (23 gold medals, 28 in all), used visualization when preparing for competition. U.S. Olympic men's swimming coach Bob Bowman described Phelps's mental rehearsal in an interview with *Forbes* in 2016: "For months before a race Michael gets into a relaxed state. He mentally rehearses for two hours a day in the pool. He sees himself winning. He smells the air, tastes the water, hears the sounds, sees the clock."[24]

Phelps would also imagine himself as a spectator in the crowd, watching the race, seeing himself overcome obstacles like falling behind. He understood that when you envision doing a task, your brain reacts as if you were physically performing it.[25] Says Bowman succinctly, "The brain can't distinguish between something that's vividly imagined and something that is real."[26]

The phenomenon of neuroplasticity helps explain why it can be so difficult to break unwanted habits, such as fearful thoughts or our favorite means of coping with stress, whether sugar binges or alcohol consumption. Those mental and physical habits developed from repetitive stress-response behaviors. They became unconscious because the brain likes to take short cuts and conserve energy for more demanding tasks, such as critical thinking or problem solving.

Think about driving a car. At first, you had to consciously think about every single step: putting the key in the ignition, turning it, shifting into gear, pressing the gas pedal or the brake. With enough practice, that all happens automatically now. How many times have you found you can't remember the last 20 minutes of your drive because you've been thinking about something else?

Or consider a dance performance, which would be unbearable for both audience and performers if the dancers had to think about each movement before they made it. (Dancers call what drives their unconscious performing *muscle memory*.) While it's useful when driving a car or performing, unconscious behavior is hardly beneficial when we're pouring another glass of wine or bingeing on Netflix with a bag of Doritos. Those life pleasures are great in moderation, but when they become habitual, they can be harmful.

And breaking that unhealthy cycle is not about "positive thinking." Yes, the brain is quite malleable and can change with concentrated thought alone. But chronic stress and years of negative emotions have created powerful connections within the brain that will take daily repetitive, physical action to change.

It starts with developing greater awareness of our thoughts and emotions. But first, we need to understand how powerful even our unconscious thoughts and beliefs can be.

The Power of Belief

Consider how a placebo works. The phenomenon known as the placebo effect occurs when a fake drug or treatment elicits a physical response, simply because the subjects *believed* they were getting an actual treatment that could help them.

An eye-opening study performed by researchers at the Baylor College of Medicine, in Houston, in 2002 demonstrates the power of placebo. Almost 200 people with painful osteoarthritis of the knee were divided into three groups, although no one knew which group he or she was in. Those in two of the groups were given a type of arthroscopic surgery; with the third, the surgeon made small incisions and took the same amount of time but removed no cartilage.

Yet *all* of the groups reported pain relief. Yes, even the people who underwent no surgery felt less pain, because they *believed* they actually had the surgery![27]

The placebo group has long been a standard part of scientific study. Recently, however, some researchers are using "open-label placebos," which means that the subjects *know* they are getting a placebo treatment. You may think that if people were aware they were getting no treatment, they would find no improvement in their symptoms. But that's not always the case.

Can you imagine going to your doctor complaining about pain, and he says, "Well, we have this drug that's just a little sugar pill, but if you believe it's going to make you feel better, it probably will"? And then it actually works? As crazy as that might sound, it has been documented.

Ted J. Kaptchuk, a professor of medicine and global health at Harvard Medical School, worked on four studies, each with more than 60 patients. In one, the participants had irritable bowel syndrome, an often-debilitating condition that causes constipation, abdominal cramping, and diarrhea. Half the study volunteers were given the open-label placebo; the others got nothing at all. The researchers found that the placebo group's symptoms improved dramatically, even though they knew they had not taken any active medication.[28]

Since the placebo group is routinely used in medical studies and clinical trials, we've long known that beliefs have a powerful influence over the brain and body. It is often our interpretation or belief about an event that affects our well-being. That accounts for the chest tightness people feel when they see their phone ringing, realize it's their boss, and react as if they are in trouble even when they haven't done anything wrong.

In the late twenties, sociologists William Isaac Thomas and Dorothy Swaine Thomas came up with the Thomas Theorem, which states that a person's interpretation of a situation can cause the outcome. In other words, the way a person subjectively thinks about a situation, or what he believes about the situation, can directly affect what follows.

This notion was based on observing a mentally ill prisoner who violently attacked fellow inmates whenever he saw them talking. Regardless of what they were saying, and without ever confronting them first, he believed they were bad-mouthing him every time they conversed. Whenever he saw this, he attacked, not because of what they were doing—because the inmates were not, in fact, discussing him—but because of what he thought they were doing.[29]

After the patient flatlined during the procedure I described earlier, it was my fear of hesitating again, with a patient's life at risk, that led to the chronic stress I carried with me for so long. It wasn't the situation itself that caused my stress, because it only happened that one time. But in my mind, it happened hundreds of times, because I had consciously created a powerful unconscious, habitual reaction.

We all hold onto beliefs and interpret life situations in ways that hurt our health: We aren't making enough money; there's not enough time in the day to get things done. These beliefs can lead to the emotions of fear, anxiety, and worry that lower our sense of well-being and can literally make us sick.[30]

I learned to reduce my stress by using my logical, conscious brain to manage my emotional, unconscious brain. It starts by being more mindful of our negative emotions, so that we can analyze them, quickly move through them, and focus our thoughts in directions that promote greater health and well-being.

Managing Stress

The first thing I did to specifically tackle my stress was to wake up earlier. As soon as I got up, I would head downstairs, sit on the couch in a comfortable position, and bury my head in a book. The reading sparked creative thinking, so I would take a few minutes to capture my ideas in a journal. Once I finished writing, I would simply close my eyes, reflect on what I had read and written, and end the routine by focusing on my breathing—taking slow, deep breaths, in and out, in and out—for 10 to 20 minutes.

Simply by concentrating on my breathing like that, I was meditating. Meditation is not a practice reserved for Tibetan monks. You don't need to sit in any particular position and "not think." Mundane activities such as walking in nature, jogging, fishing, even cutting the grass can put us into a relaxed, almost euphoric state. I found that meditating enhanced my focus and concentration, calmed my emotions, and gave me a greater sense of peace. It helped lower my heart rate and blood pressure and put my brain waves into that twilight, semiconscious theta state.

It wasn't long before I started meditating in the middle of the day or right before I got home. About a mile away from my house, I would pull over and park in a corner of a restaurant parking lot, close my eyes, and concentrate on my breathing, the same way I did in the morning. That peaceful 10 minutes could clear away all the chaos of the day. It was like hitting a reset button on my brain.

It's no surprise that not bringing my work stress home with me made me a better father and husband. I wasn't as emotionally drained when I got home. I had higher levels of energy. And instead of being on my phone so much of the time, working and worrying about the next day, I was more engaged with my family.

Through meditating, I developed the self-awareness to note when I felt like a ticking time bomb, and I learned how to defuse it. That self-awareness, also referred to as mindfulness, helped me lessen the stress response throughout the day.

Mindfulness is nothing more than being present in the moment: being aware of our thoughts and feelings here and now; noticing what is going on around us and inside us; observing the world without judgment. Mindfulness is essentially using our logical brain to observe and analyze the effects of our emotional brain. It has been practiced for thousands of years in many cultures.

Countless scientific studies have shown that a consistent daily meditation practice lowers stress, improves focus and self-control, and increases self-awareness.[31] When compared with the reactions of non-meditators, it reduces the rise in cortisol during stressful events. It can enlarge the brain areas involved in emotional regulation and even increase one's overall sense of happiness.

Jon Kabat Zinn, PhD, a molecular biologist, developed a practice combining meditation, self-awareness, and yoga that he calls Mindfulness-Based Stress Reduction. It has been used for decades in clinical settings for pain management and various stress-related life issues.

Recall that stress decreases activity in the prefrontal cortex, the part of the brain responsible for conscious thought and planning, while increasing activity in the amygdala. In one study, led by Harvard-affiliated researchers at Massachusetts General Hospital in 2010, 16 "meditation-naive" subjects took an eight-week-long MBSR program at the University of Massachusetts Center for Mindfulness. MRI images taken before they started and after they finished indicated "changes in gray matter concentration in brain regions involved in learning and memory processes, emotion regulation, self-referential processing, and perspective taking."[32]

In other words, the MRI scans showed that the amygdala (in the emotional, fight-or-flight part of the brain) appeared to shrink and the prefrontal cortex (part of the logical brain) became thicker. Yes, this study showed that a consistent meditative practice diminished the part of the brain involved in stressful emotions and enlarged the part involved in logical thinking. Other research has shown that meditation strengthens the connection between these two brain regions.[33] All of these benefits simply from being more self-aware! I can't swear that's what happened in my brain, but it sure seems that was the case.

In addition to my morning and after-work routines, I used mindfulness at work in the operating room, especially during procedures where patients' hearts were in vulnerable situations. Any time fearful memories of a patient flatlining would creep back into my head, I would consciously tell myself that I was prepared and that I'd be fine. I would take slow, deep breaths. I would stand up straight, with my chin up and my chest out slightly.

I felt so much more at ease when I shifted my posture to a confident pose and breathed more slowly. When we breathe, our heart rate changes a bit: When we inhale, it increases slightly, and when we exhale, it decreases slightly. This is known as Respiratory Sinus Arrhythmia.[34] When we take control of our breathing and consciously exhale slowly, we can significantly slow our heart rate down. That alone helps us relax.

Yoga practitioners and monks have used breathing practices for centuries to relax their minds and control their emotions. Typical unconscious breathing patterns involve shallow inhalations in the upper chest. A more beneficial way to breathe is to consciously inhale deeply into the belly, which fills the lungs in their entirety. Taking such deep breaths oxygenates the blood, which may increase the production of serotonin, endorphins, and dopamine.[35]

And taking deep breaths affects the sympathetic nervous system, which is the mechanism in control of the fight-or-flight response. Deep breathing triggers the opposing mechanism, the parasympathetic nervous system, which inhibits it.[36]

I also consciously shifted my attention to something more positive, like my wife and my kids. Distraction from the stress expedited my response to it.

Mindfulness helped me break the cycle of cookie bingeing, too. Because I was so in tune with my emotions now, I knew right away when the sugar craving was about to hit. When that happened, I would ask my wife to hide the Oreos. (How pathetic, I know—but I needed help, and it worked!) I started eating grapes instead. They satisfied my sweet tooth and were a much healthier option.

Thanks to my meditation routine, I was far less stressed, so the cravings themselves diminished dramatically. They didn't disappear, but when they would arise, I was ready for them. Of course, I wasn't able to prevent all negative emotions from occurring in my life—I doubt that's even possible!—but I was able to manage them with my logical brain.

Though the kind of meditation I practice most is mindfulness meditation, I began experimenting with other types of meditation as well: gratitude, loving-kindness, and mental imagery. I will describe all these stress-reducing practices—breathing and posture, visualization, journaling, various types of meditation, and more, in Part 3.

Part 2: Philosophy - Purpose, Meaning and Happiness

Perception vs. Reality

I believe the way to truly overcome our self-inflicted chronic stress is to fundamentally change the way we think about the world. It took me a little while to realize that.

I had developed a consistent habit of meditation and was more mindful of my feelings throughout the day. I was using these techniques to calm my emotions, curb my sugar cravings, and stop perpetuating the stress response. I was sleeping better, was happier at home and more productive at work, because I had learned how to manage my stress, those fearful feelings I had developed way back in college. While I was better equipped to deal with the emotional responses that resulted from the fear, I was still unable to eliminate my chronic fear itself.

I still worried about failure, about letting people down, and—now that I was older—about making enough money, paying the bills, even putting my kids through college. I know; people in a far worse situation would love to have these "First World" problems. But no matter how much I tried to tell myself that, the fear still dominated. In my experience, it doesn't matter if you are rich or poor, healthy or sick, happy or depressed. Fear can always be present in some capacity.

Because I was so afraid of failure and so concerned with what others thought, I was still a "yes man" and a people pleaser, overwhelmed with trying to make people happy all the time. I developed a habit of sweating the small things. Going to the grocery store became a big ordeal, because of my fearful thinking. Do I have enough time to get there? What was I supposed to pick up again? What if I forget something?

This is the way my mind was operating all the time. I even worried about buying my grapes: If I don't get to the store today or they're out, what am I going to eat if I get a sugar craving?

Thankfully, through mindfulness meditation I was more self-aware, and I came to the realization that I needed to change the way I viewed the world. To generate more positive actions and emotions, I needed to replace my negative thinking with positive thinking. Just as I had changed my brain, I needed to change my mind.

I started to wonder: If I want to reduce my fear, which causes my stress, and live a fuller life, where should I direct my thoughts? Beyond focusing on basic tasks—raising a family well, doing my best at my job, being a good husband and supportive friend, living in a healthy, productive way—what should I set my mind *on*? Naturally, I started thinking about things that made me happy. What I soon realized was that my *perceived* source of happiness actually didn't make me happy at all.

Three Degrees of Happiness

People who are just trying to survive don't have time to think about happiness. And it probably makes sense that in this and other wealthy countries, people are obsessed with making money, because they think it will make them happy. When I first entered the workforce, I focused on making as much money as I could, because it made me happy! I loved pursuing and thinking about it.

Having lots of money would mean I could have a really nice car, an expensive watch, fashionable clothes, go out to good restaurants, and show the world that I was successful. Having a lot of money would mean I could buy gifts for my wife and awesome toys for my kids. All those things could and did bring *temporary* happiness, but it inevitably faded. And thinking about money turned out to bring more stress than joy.

When I became more mindful of my money-focused mindset, I realized that when I earned more money, the fear of having less became that much worse. I was plagued with thoughts like "What if I lost my job? There's no way I could find another job and make this much money right away. I'd have to start at the bottom and work my way up again. That would be 10 years down the drain.... I need to make more now so that I'll have a bigger security blanket in case the market tanks and I get laid off.... Maybe I could move into another division? But I worked really hard to get good at the pacemaker job. What if I don't do well in a new position and make less money, or they let me go?"

These were the kinds of thoughts that would fill my head. Sure, getting that bonus filled me with joy for a few days, but then the fear would set in again. I just pushed through it as I always had, because the money was what mattered. For years, I was on this relentless pursuit of what I thought would bring me happiness.

Research confirms what I came to realize. In the long run, many things that people think will make them happy do not, and money is one of those things. A 2010 study out of Princeton University's Woodrow Wilson School of Public and International Affairs found there's no significant increase in happiness for people in the U.S. who make over $75,000 a year. Angus Deaton, an economist, and Daniel Kahneman, a psychologist who won a Nobel Prize for Economics, analyzed the responses of 450,000 Americans polled in 2008 and 2009. In addition to income, the participants were asked how they had felt the previous day and if they believed they were living the best possible life.

According to the reporting in *Time* magazine, the researchers found that most Americans (85 percent) feel happy each day regardless of annual income, but that the lower it fell below $75,000, the more their problems wore away at them. Those who made about $75,000 a year or more (in 2010, remember) were more affected by temperament and life circumstances—illness or divorce, say—than by how much money they brought home.[1]

In fact, as an article in the *New York Times* in 2006 noted, "In recent years, researchers have reported an ever-growing list of downsides to getting and spending." These included "damage to relationships and self-esteem, a heightened risk of depression and anxiety, [and] less time for what the research indicates truly makes people happy, like family, friendship and engaging work."[2]

So why do people value money so much? Yes, it may bring freedom, security, the ability to acquire more things, but don't we yearn for those things because we assume they'll make us happy? Aristotle said that happiness is the one thing we desire in and of itself.[3]

It is "the meaning and the purpose of life, the whole aim and end of human existence."[4]

Indulging in tasty food and drink, buying a big house, an expensive car, lots of clothing or jewelry, getting the best seats at a ballgame or an opera or a play.... All these things may give pleasure in the short term and can be great in moderation. But we all know that none of them brings long-term happiness.

For me, pleasure came mostly from money (and sweets to combat my stress). But my wife and kids didn't need the things I bought for them; they just needed me. And not the me who was always on his phone working. They needed the me who was fully present and experiencing life with them, there in that precious moment.

A source of happiness closely related to *materialistic pleasures*—tangible objects such as money, cars, homes—is what Robert J. Spitzer, PhD, calls *comparative pleasures*: celebrity or fame, status, "keeping up with the Joneses." In *Finding True Happiness: Satisfying Our Restless Hearts*, Spitzer, a Jesuit priest, offers a chart describing four levels of happiness, rooted in Aristotelian thinking. Materialistic and comparative pleasures are listed on the first and second levels.[5]

Comparative pleasures, which have everything to do with ego, build on materialism. It's so easy to get caught up in trying to bolster our egos and find happiness through materialistic sources, because society is constantly driving us to do just that. Think of all the commercials, ads, billboards, and social media we come across each day, encouraging us to spend our money on something a celebrity is promoting, or to buy something *everyone* has and do something *everyone* is doing. It's maddening, and I often succumbed to those constant pressures.

Once I purchased a fancy SUV, a Yukon Denali. It had all the bells and whistles you can imagine: big rims, heated leather seats, heads-up display, DVD player, Apple car play—the works. I have always loved big, expensive vehicles. People weren't driving around in cars like that in the small town I grew up in, so it was always a big deal to see one, and an even bigger deal to own one. I mean, come on; that's one of the reasons I got into medical sales—to make good money so I could afford things like that car. It is why I pushed harder and harder through the stress and adversity, to hit the sales numbers and be successful.

Since I was making good money, I was able to buy a big, expensive Denali that I didn't need. But boy, did I want it, and boy, did it feel good to drive it off the lot! In my mind, it showed how successful I was. That new-car smell, the comfort, the smooth ride, the feeling of owning the road—lots of dopamine reactions in the brain from that bad boy!

Yes, I did feel great driving that SUV around. But the joy that vehicle brought me faded after about two weeks, and I was left with a very expensive lesson in happiness. It doesn't come from acquiring things.

Spitzer calls his third level of happiness, after the materialistic and comparative, *contributive pleasures*. They come from family, friends, being a part of social or religious organizations, involvement in charitable activities.

Here we move on from *things* (cars, fashion) and *ego* (how people perceive us) to *action*: taking care of our families, being a good friend, getting involved in activities we care about, and helping others. That last one can be as simple as stopping to hold the door for someone or as involved as providing care for someone who is sick. I was actually doing that in my work but had been too blinded by fear and stress to see how impactful and giving my job was.

The body can't be in a state of fear and a state of compassion at the same time. Once I began doing more of the little things (like holding the door) for others, I noticed my fearful thoughts begin to dissipate and felt greater satisfaction in my own life. That led to more contributive action, like playing with my kids more, doing more around the house—little things that can have a big impact—and donating to charities instead of buying something.

Purpose and Meaning

In addition to giving me real happiness, these little acts began to bring a renewed sense of meaning and purpose to my life. I've come to believe that this is what people truly desire.

"Life is never made unbearable by circumstances," Viktor E. Frankl wrote in *Man's Search for Meaning*, "but only by lack of meaning and purpose."[6] Frankl, a psychotherapist who had studied with Freud, wrote this after surviving not one but several concentration camps. (Originally published in 1946, his book is still in print and is assigned reading in many schools.) Frankl found that once his fellow prisoners lost their sense of purpose, they lost their will to live and tended to sicken and die. He even wrote, "In some ways suffering ceases to be suffering at the moment it finds a meaning, such as the meaning of a sacrifice."[7]

The pressure to make more money and the fear of not hitting my sales numbers seemed completely absurd when I thought about people who had far greater challenges in life. For example, people in poor health—like those I was encountering every day! When I thought about the joy I brought to patients after telling them, "Your device just saved your life," I suddenly wasn't so plagued by stress and fear. In fact, I felt grateful for having the ability to help others.

Instead of rushing off to the next hospital and the next procedure, I took the time to offer kind words and interact with each patient. I consciously focused on their questions and needs and spent more time with them. I could tell I had changed when I started getting more compliments on my bedside manner, and more comments on how much I had helped, than I'd ever had in my life.

Later, I found greater purpose in my life by writing this book. Things that used to annoy me—waking up early, driving to and from work, "wasted" time when a procedure was delayed—became some of the most productive parts of my day, because I used that time to create and organize material for the book. I took the money I'd normally spend on fancy toys like the Denali and put it to better use in creating this book and a platform to help others with their health.

At home, I started talking to my wife in a more intimate way, to find out how I could best help her, and took action to make it a reality. I put the phone away and gave my kids my full attention, playing with greater energy, thanks to my meditation routine. By simply giving more of myself to the people in my life, I was able to better appreciate the real sources of meaning and purpose in life.

That gave me more incentive to eat better and even find time to exercise more. Research shows that when we have a sense of purpose, we tend to take better care of ourselves. An article in the *Journal of Health Psychology* first published in 2014 described a study in which, after completing "measures of purpose in life," volunteers wore accelerometers for three consecutive days. The researchers found purpose in life "positively associated with objectively measured movement, moderate to vigorous physical activity, and with self-reported activity."[8]

Another study, at Flinders University in Adelaide, Australia, and reported in *Psychology Today* in 2015, looked at 1,475 older adults who were part of the Australian Longitudinal Study of Aging. They had cognitive abilities (short-term memory and mental speed) tested and answered questions on their health history, depression, how they viewed their health, and the goals they wished to achieve. Over the course of 18 years, the subjects were interviewed four more times. The researchers found that having a strong sense of purpose correlated with fewer symptoms of depression, lower functional disability, better cognitive abilities, and better "self-rated" health. Survival analysis indicated that having a strong sense of purpose was also related to living longer, although this became less apparent over time as the subjects aged.[9]

More recently, a 2019 study, published in *JAMA Current Open* and described on the National Public Radio website *Shots: Health News From NPR*, found that people who lacked what the researchers called "a self-organizing life aim that stimulates goals" were more than twice as likely to die as those who had a life purpose. Specifically, they were more likely to die of cardiovascular diseases. This held true regardless of the subjects' gender, race, level of education, and economic status.

The information came from more than 7,000 American adults. They were not asked about how they found meaning in their lives, just how powerful they felt it was. And get this: It appears that having a life purpose has more effect on decreasing your risk of death than exercising regularly or drinking or smoking less.

One of the authors of the study told NPR, "I approached this with a very skeptical eye." Celeste Leigh Pearce, PhD, is associate chair and an associate professor of epidemiology at the University of Michigan, in Ann Arbor. She found the results so convincing, "I'm developing a whole research program around it."

Alan Rozanski, M.D., a professor at the Icahn School of Medicine at Mount Sinai, in New York, was not involved in this project but has studied the relationship between life purpose and health. He agrees with Viktor Frankl: "The need for meaning and purpose is No. 1. It's the deepest driver of well-being there is."[10]

Pursuing a purpose in life might improve longevity because of its effect on telomeres, those caps at the ends of the strings of chromosomes that contain our DNA. Elizabeth Blackburn, PhD, professor emeritus in the department of biochemistry and biophysics at the University of California, San Francisco, won the 2009 Nobel Prize for Physiology or Medicine for her research into telomeres, specifically relating to psychological stress and physical aging. She shares the credit for discovering an enzyme called telomerase, which slows that process.

Because of the damage to the telomeres, which can lead to sickness and poor longevity, Blackburn knew that people with chronic stress tend to have shortened chromosomes. She was part of a study that looked at two major contributors to stress, neuroticism and "perceived control," as well as at telomerase activity. In a study reported in the journal *Psychoneuroendocrinology* in 2011, participants joined a three-month retreat during which they meditated six hours a day. Compared to a control group, they showed more "telomerase activity," greater perceived control, and less neuroticism. In addition, "increases in both mindfulness and purpose in life" were greater in the retreat group.[11]

When he examined this study, Victor J. Strecher, PhD, a professor of health behavior and health education at the University of Michigan School of Public Health, concluded that meditating had helped create a greater sense of purpose—that having a purpose in life, not meditation itself, was related to the increased telomerase activity.[12]

Strecher wrote about Blackburn's work in his book *Life on Purpose: How Living for What Matters Most Changes Everything*. His book cites a study showing that with every one-point increase on a scale measuring purpose in life, adults with heart disease decreased their chances of a heart attack by 27 percent.[13] Another study indicated that students who felt their education was relevant to their life purpose were more likely to work hard in classes they found difficult or boring.[14]

Transcendent Happiness

Materialistic and ego-centered pleasures are fleeting, not a true source of fulfillment. Charity and doing things for others is certainly a component and a good start. But the greatest degree of happiness, the icing on the cake for me in terms of my purpose and new mindset, comes from what Robert Spitzer puts on his fourth and highest level of happiness: *transcendent pleasures.*

This level builds on contributive happiness but goes far beyond being more loving, compassionate, and giving. It has to do with what Spitzer describes as the pursuit of perfect truth, beauty, goodness, and love.

Seeking *truth* means using our minds or intellect to explore, to think critically and logically, to use science to advance our understanding of the world so that we can better it. Beyond that, it means filling our minds with thoughts of love and goodness, which trigger virtuous action.

That's a lot, I know. Let's start with the pursuit of truth or, if you like, of knowledge. In a 2012 post on her blog, cognitive neuroscientist Caroline Leaf, PhD, author of *Switch on Your Brain: The Key to Peak Happiness, Thinking and Health*, wrote, "The deeper you think the more intelligent you become. The deeper you think the more thoughts and memories you will grow inside your brain. We are not designed to skim the surface of things, but rather to think things through, to read deeply, to understand and build strong memories."[15]

Citing a study led by Dr. Katrina Walsemann of the University of South Carolina Arnold School of Public Health, she added, "The deep pursuit of knowledge increases not only our intelligence but also our health." This study looked at individuals who were part of the National Longitudinal Survey of Youth 1979. Attaining at least a bachelor's degree by age 25 was associated with fewer depressive symptoms and better self-rated health when compared with respondents who did not attain a higher degree by midlife.[16]

Beauty comes in many forms: art, music, poetry and literature, nature, even, through the miracle of childbirth, a new human life. Being mindful of beauty means being fully present in the moment—not stressing over the past or worrying about the future but taking in the here and now—focusing on what is going on around us in all its glory and cherishing each precious moment we are alive.

When we're lucky, that can lead to awe. A study from the University of California, Irvine, described in the *Journal of Personality and Social Psychology* in 2015 found that experiencing awe, "that sense of wonder we feel in the presence of something vast that transcends our understanding of the world," promotes altruism and loving-kindness. In one part of the study, the researchers placed participants amid a grove of towering eucalyptus trees and found a correlation between their feelings of awe and what the researchers called prosocial (positive, helpful, and friendly) behavior.

As Paul Piff, a member of the research team, wrote, "By diminishing the emphasis on the individual self, awe may encourage people to forgo strict self-interest to improve the welfare of others. When experiencing awe, you may not, egocentrically speaking, feel like you're at the center of the world anymore."[17]

Goodness means directing something toward its ultimate purpose; putting others first; being empathetic; developing deep, meaningful relationships. As I found out, that has personal benefits! "Doing Good Does You Good," a post on the Mental Health Foundation website, notes that forms of altruism, including volunteering, mentoring, doing work for a good cause, and performing random acts of kindness, can lead to a reduction in stress and negative feelings, a sense of belonging, improved physical health, even a longer life.[18]

Love and goodness go hand in hand. According to one of the greatest philosophers in history, Thomas Aquinas, love is simply willing the good of another. This in and of itself is beautiful. And anyone who's been in love knows how good it makes you feel. According to Helen Riess, M.D., associate clinical professor of psychiatry at Harvard Medical School, director of the Empathy and Relational Science Program at Massachusetts General Hospital, and author of *The Empathy Effect*, love releases dopamine, a feel-good chemical. Later, another brain chemical, oxytocin, or "the bonding hormone," kicks in. Being in a loving relationship can ease loneliness and anxiety, help you stay healthier, and even live longer.[19]

Living a Transcendent Life

I think we can all agree with Dr. Spitzer that living a materialistic, ego-centered, or even contributive life would not be as satisfying in the long term as one with a focus on the transcendent: truth, beauty, goodness, love. How often have we heard of people living a life of service and charity, love and gratitude going back to materialistic ways? Never, in my experience. But there are plenty of stories out there of people who have all the money in the world and are miserable.

I was fortunate to have a friend and mentor who was just the opposite: extremely successful and yet living a life of true fulfillment. His name is Jim. He was born and raised in the same town I was. As a running back at our high school, he set legendary records that stood for decades, until the running back on the team I played on broke them. (This was big news in our little hometown, where Friday night football was a very big deal.) Jim left when he got a scholarship to play college football.

Though I knew a lot about him, I had never met him, so I was excited to learn years later that Jim was living near the town I live in now. Always interested in networking, I looked him up and found that he was quite willing to help someone from his hometown further his career. I can't tell you how much he taught me through the years of our friendship about business, sales, marketing.... But he taught me far more about how to live a good life.

Jim went out of his way to make me feel welcome whenever I visited him. He was always interested in how I was doing, what he could do to help me, how to make my day a little better. He frequently expressed his love for the people in his life, including me. Beyond that, he had a genuine interest in people.

I will never forget the time we were driving back from lunch and were sitting at a stoplight. He was in the passenger seat. It was a warm, sunny day, so we had the windows down; the car in the next lane had its windows down, too. Out of the blue, he started talking with the driver, a complete stranger. After a few seconds, it sounded as if they had known each other for years.

What I found most surprising about this simple, brief encounter was that just as the light turned green, Jim said, "Praise the Lord on this beautiful day!" And the other person shouted, "Amen, my brother!" I was blown away by this exchange. It was the first time outside my adolescent churchgoing days that I had heard expressions of faith in a public setting between two people who didn't even know each other. I actually felt a little awkward.

But Jim wasn't shy about sharing his deep thoughts and faith with the people he came in contact with. In our conversations about business and career paths, we always ended up talking about life, love, family and relationships, meaning and purpose. Jim got me to really start thinking about the big life questions: Why am I here? What am I supposed to do with my time on earth? What is the meaning of life? What happens after I die, if anything? For Jim, the ultimate source of purpose and meaning was God.

I had been raised Catholic by deeply religious parents and gone to Catholic grade school, but I hadn't attended church regularly or thought deeply about religion or God in a long time. I had become so entrenched in doing my job and raising a family that I had no time for anything else. Especially the nonsense of religion. I mean, come on; I worked in the medical field. Religion is all about fairy tales and miracles. I've seen what real medicine and innovative technology can do for people.

Do you think it's reasonable to believe there's a magical old man in the sky who is running the show? Growing up, I believed in God, the Bible, and my school teachings because that's what I was told to believe. You could say my faith was blind, because I had never looked into it.

After many conversations with Jim, I decided to do that. For years, I researched scientific and philosophical explanations for the existence of the universe, for the ultimate source of meaning, purpose, and life. I consumed countless books, audiobooks, podcasts, and YouTube videos from various perspectives and belief systems. I stumbled upon some of the greatest philosophers in history, and the way they thought about reality completely blew my mind! The logic and rationality they used to describe the source of life was something I had never encountered before, and even more surprising, it made complete sense to me.

My philosophical thinking and research led me to (re)adopt the belief that there actually is a fundamental source of reality—of all that exists—which created it and sustains it right now, in this very moment. Whether we choose to call it a universal consciousness, an ultimate power, an infinite intelligence, or simply God is irrelevant. The nature or characteristics of this source is what's important.

This source, by definition, *is* perfect love, perfect goodness, perfect truth, and perfect beauty. These cannot be measured. They are not grounded in nature or our brains. They transcend this world and are the ultimate source of happiness, because they are transcendent aspects of reality.

Believing that this source exists doesn't mean that an all-powerful deity is pulling the strings, that we aren't in control of our lives, so it doesn't matter what we do. I believe that this higher power—let's just call it God—gave us love, goodness, beauty, logic, free will, and the consciousness that makes us uniquely human.

We are in charge of the way we act. We can freely choose to be better. We have the rational capabilities to improve ourselves and to influence others through our thoughts and actions, specifically pertaining to goodness and love.

Anselm of Canterbury, a philosopher, Benedictine monk, and the archbishop of Canterbury (1093-1109), said, "God is that which nothing greater can be thought."[20] If I wanted to change the way I viewed the world to the greatest possible degree, why not focus on that than which nothing greater can be thought? (For anyone interested in how I came to agree with the philosophical arguments for the existence and nature of God—to feel it is rational to believe that God is the fundamental source of existence, and that this particular belief can lead to greater well-being—check out the Appendix.)

If you felt you had a better sense of the answers to life's big questions, or even a glimmer of the answers leading to greater meaning and purpose, wouldn't you feel happier? Why not *try* to see the world through the lens of perfect love, goodness, beauty, and truth?

We Can Choose How We View the World

I chose to adopt the notion that if God exists, then this life is not all there is, and that ultimately, pain and suffering will cease to exist—that perfect love, perfect goodness, perfect beauty, and perfect truth will be realized in some way after we die. Though pain and suffering are a part of life, that does not have to define or hamper our lives. We can manage pain and suffering with our rational capabilities. We have the ability to use our minds to interpret things that happen to us.

We can choose love and goodness, even in times of great distress. And we can reframe the way we view evil. Though he experienced some of the worst evils in human history, Dr. Frankl was able to create a great book that illustrates that notion. In *Man's Search for Meaning*, he wrote, "Forces beyond your control can take away everything you possess except one thing, your freedom to choose how you will respond to the situation. You cannot control what happens to you in life, but you can always control what you will feel and do about what happens to you."[21] Human beings have the freedom to choose their thoughts, Frankl says, and to change in any instance.[22]

This way of thinking has helped me enormously in dealing with the day-to-day stresses and sources of fear in my life. One example is the daily news. If you pay any attention to the headlines, you see constant examples of death, destruction, people hurting themselves, people hurting one another—just reading some of the stories, especially about children, would trigger a stress response. But with greater self-awareness, I was able to recognize when I was getting worked up. My new optimistic mindset and some rationality helped me eliminate the news as a source of stress and fear.

Take, for example, any of the stories about gun violence. While these are, of course, absolutely tragic and emotionally brutal, I tried to understand, from a logical perspective, why so many of these instances were occurring, as well as why the media were putting them front and center. And I tried to understand the humanity of the shooters. They might be in terrible pain themselves and, in the heat of the moment, perhaps had little control over their emotions. While this certainly doesn't justify their actions, it helps me process them.

Though the overload of terrible news encourages us to think otherwise, I still cling to the idea (well, it's more of a hope) that the majority of society is not bad.

As for all those headlines centered on violence and death, remember that our emotional brains encode the negative more strongly than the positive to keep us from potential danger by activating the stress response.[23] Eventually, I used my logical brain to overcome that emotional urge to keep paying attention and cut back on how much news I consume. The news I choose to follow is more uplifting in nature, and when I come across something negative, I try to find a more compassionate way of processing it.

From Frankl once more: "When we are no longer able to change a situation, we are challenged to change ourselves."[24]

Divine Empathy

I found that the process of critical thinking and rationalizing my position within the universe brought me great joy. Human beings are unique in that regard. Not only are we able to ponder our existence and control our outlook on life, we can strengthen those abilities. We can attain a greater level of happiness through the self-awareness, empathy, compassion, intelligence, creativity, and virtuous actions that make us genuine human beings.

Whether or not you believe in a higher power, you can choose to pretend you are God, or to act like God, by reflecting God's divine attributes. Call it divine empathy. You can pursue truth with your logical mind. You can focus on and create beauty. You can consistently will the good of others and live a virtuous life. That doesn't mean never making a mistake or not ever hurting anyone; it means always trying to do the right thing. It means pursuing perfection. Of course, you will fail, often. And others will fail you, but that's okay. We are all far from perfect. But we can consciously try to be better.

That's why it is so important to forgive. Forgiveness is a part of transcendent happiness, but it is also one of the most difficult actions to achieve, because when someone wrongs us, it hurts. When a loved one lies to us or someone steals from us, the urge to get back at them is powerful. But we are rational beings. We can put ourselves in other people's shoes and try to understand why they made the choices they did. We can use our logical brain to overcome strong emotions, employ empathy, and forgive.

And forgiveness should be bestowed on ourselves as well as on others, particularly when we're trying to overcome chronic fearful thoughts and actions. Why? In addition to the philosophical reasons, forgiveness—yes, you guessed it—is good for our health!

Research suggests that forgiveness has a positive effect on blood pressure, sleep, immune function, and stress. In a study published in the *Journal of Health Psychology* in 2014, 148 young adults were asked to assess their lifetime stress levels, their tendency to forgive, and their overall mental and physical health. Those with more exposure to stress were, no surprise, in poorer health physically and mentally. Interestingly, however, the researchers found that with those who were more forgiving of both themselves and others, the link between stress and mental illness was almost eliminated.[25]

"It's almost entirely erased—it's statistically zero," Loren Toussaint, an associate professor of psychology at Luther College, in Decorah, Iowa, and one of the study's authors, told a reporter for *Time* magazine. "If you don't have forgiving tendencies, you feel the raw effects of stress in an unmitigated way. You don't have a buffer against that stress." Toussaint says he believes "100 percent" that forgiveness can be learned. "I think most people want to feel good and [forgiveness] offers you the opportunity to do that."[26]

As Viktor Frankl wrote, "Everything can be taken from a man but one thing: the last of the human freedoms—to choose one's attitude in any given set of circumstances, to choose one's own way."[27] That is to say, we have the freedom to turn the other cheek, to reach out to someone who has hurt us, to forgive, to love.

When you look at the world through the lens of perfect love and goodness, it's easier to see the other person's point of view. Your stress diminishes, because you're in a positive, loving state.

Every interaction with other human beings is an opportunity to improve our own lives, as well as theirs. I realized greater meaning and purpose simply through going deeper with my words and actions, even toward complete strangers, like my friend Jim—being kinder, more empathetic, more selfless, more loving—things I should have been doing all along but had never even considered, because of my stress and fear.

Communication Is Key

I didn't forget to take better action toward the people closest to me, either. I can't tell you how many times my wife and I had fallen into the trap of acting more like roommates or coworkers while I was going through a stressful period. We would hardly talk; not because we didn't want to or were mad at each other, but because we were busy with two demanding full-time jobs and three kids under five years old. At the end of the day, I was simply too exhausted to have any kind of meaningful conversation. I was usually preoccupied with my phone or my work, anyway.

When my mindset changed, and I started taking action toward perfect love and goodness, I began taking a more genuine interest in *her* emotional state, in the things *she* was struggling with. I did my best to figure out what would ease that stress and offer words and actions to help. While I wasn't always successful, I noticed a change in both of us. We were clicking again, like when we were first married: smiling and laughing more, feeling close, more playful with the kids, more coordinated around the house.

The funny thing is, the number one thing we did to improve our emotional states was simply to talk. Not the usual small talk after work, but the deep kind of conversation that elicited and dissected our struggles and fears.

Over time, I was better able to describe my feelings and understand hers. At first it was really hard and uncomfortable for me. Maybe it shouldn't have been, but I have never been one to open up about my feelings or dive into the feelings of others, even my wife's. And I was so busy and scatterbrained throughout the day that there had been no time for feelings. So I had to make some time.

Every once in a while, in bed right before falling asleep, we would have a very deep, meaningful conversation. Once I got used to it, it was so refreshing to bring out things that had been on our minds. There would be a noticeable change in our interactions in the following days. As soon as I recognized this cyclical pattern, I wanted to expand on it.

I came up with a perhaps cheesy yet surprisingly successful method to make our deep conversations habitual. I called it our TEE time:

T = Thought
E = Emotion
E = Experience

I love golf and over the years have had my fair share of tee times with the boys. Now I was able to have tee times with my wife. And honestly, the tee times with her are just as good as, and in many instances better than, the ones at the golf course.

The *thought* has to be something deep or philosophical, or a profound realization pertaining to our relationship or daily lives. It can come from asking questions and listening to the answers. Not the usual glib "how ya doin' today?" but "How are you really feeling? Why? What caused it? Could this have contributed? Is there anything I can do to help?"

The *emotion* can be generated from the thought shared or your response ("I felt the same way about a similar situation") or simply by coming from a loving place of compassion and encouragement. The *experience* can be anything from a hug to a surprise dinner date.

The purpose of the tee time is to consciously make an effort to connect and communicate. Rather than simply coexisting and trying to get through the day, we work to generate more one-on-one time in an intimate, face-to-face setting.

Speaking openly, honestly, and face to face with another individual seems to be a lost art today, with everyone's heads buried in their smartphones. And yes, you can have a good talk with someone over the phone, but you'll never see the many nonverbal cues exchanged during any conversation. Our body language and the expressions on our faces convey what we are truly thinking and feeling, even if our words say something different.

The importance of opening up to someone on a daily basis

cannot be overstated. But sometimes you need more help with an emotional or mental problem than a friend or loved one can give. In that case, I strongly recommend talking with a professional.

A common term for this is talk therapy, also known as psychoanalysis. It is based on the notion that we need to uncover, understand, and release the repressed emotions, thoughts, or experiences that are causing our stress and pain. But many, perhaps most, of us don't need to discover the underlying causes of our stress as much as we need to change the ways we think and act. We don't need to look into the past as much as we need to identify current unhealthy thoughts and beliefs and *change* them.

A specific form of talk therapy called Cognitive Behavioral Therapy focuses on just that. CBT involves talking with a professional and developing new ways of thinking; for instance, through mindfulness techniques and affirmations.[28]

A study in a journal called *Translational Psychiatry* and reported in *Forbes* in 2017 indicated that CBT can cause a measurable increase in neural connectivity between the amygdala (in the limbic brain, remember, thus related to fear and memory) and areas in the prefrontal cortex that govern higher-order thinking and executive function (just like meditation can!).

The participants—all of whom had been diagnosed with schizophrenia—had been in an earlier study with the same research team. All continued to take their regular medication, but some underwent CBT sessions as well. When brain scans taken before the study began and at the end of six months were compared, only those who had the CBT showed structural changes in their brain. This went on for eight years. The study found that the stronger the connectivity between these brain regions, the more people's symptoms improved over the long term.[29]

CBT can also be self-administered—that is, without the aid of a professional. Jonathan Moran describes many good techniques to combat stress and fearful thinking in his book *Cognitive Behavioral Therapy and Dialectical Behavior Therapy for Anxiety: Everything You Should Know About Treating Depression, Worry, Panic, PTSD, Phobias and Other Anxiety Symptoms with CBT & DBT.*

One example involves scheduling in writing something that you enjoy doing; focusing on that activity in the days or weeks leading up to it; and making sure you do it. This helps focus your thoughts on something positive in the future.[30] Other techniques include mindfulness (of course!), journaling, affirmations, and "cognitive restructuring," or analyzing negative thoughts and asking logical questions that will lead to new conclusions. I describe all these techniques and more in Part 3.

So many of life's stresses can be mitigated or eliminated simply by communicating with another. Keeping negative emotions trapped inside can eat away at us, especially when the things that are bothering us relate to another person. Communicating in a loving manner, in addition to virtuous acts of goodness, leads to thriving relationships.

Relationships

Powerful relationships with loved ones absolutely crush stress and fear. When my wife and I are firing on all cylinders—talking deeply, energized, helping each other with daily tasks, fully present with each other and our kids, romantic—everything in my life is better. The stress and fear are so much easier to manage, because she helps put me into a more positive state of mind.

Countless books I've read and content I've consumed confirm that the number one thing that we can do to better our lives is to focus on our relationships. Think about that for a second: All it takes to go from where you are right now to where you want to be, whether that pertains to your health, finances, job, or family, is at least one meaningful relationship.

One group of researchers who reviewed 148 studies—data about almost 309,000 individuals followed for an average of 7.5 years—found that those with "adequate" social relationships had a 50 percent greater likelihood of survival than those with insufficient or poor relationships. "The magnitude of this effect," the researchers wrote in their study, published in *PLOS Medicine* in 2010, "is comparable with quitting smoking and it exceeds many well-known risk factors for mortality (e.g., obesity, physical inactivity)." In other words, having loved ones, family, and friends in your life is really good for your health![31]

You don't have to be attractive to be someone's best friend; you don't have to be smart to be loving; you don't have to be a good athlete to really listen to someone and offer support; you don't have to be talented to be kind. Just as we are rational, we are also relational beings. Improve your relationship with your higher power, improve your relationship with those closest to you, improve your relationship with yourself, and you will reduce your stress, be happier, perhaps even live longer.

I can think of no better example of realizing greater meaning and purpose through relationships—in fact, of transcendent fulfillment—than fatherhood. Being a father, but more specifically, being *mindful* of fatherhood, has taught me more about myself and about life than I could have ever imagined. It's so simple, yet so profound: We have been gifted with the ability to create and influence human life. By choosing to have children, I chose not only to create but to make my first concern the growth and the good of another human being.

I took this for granted at first, too blind to see that the answers to my big "life questions" were right there in front of me, in the form of my family. For years, I had had great purpose and meaning in my life but hardly recognized it, because of my stress and fear.

Another word for relationship is *love*. The pursuit of love leads to powerful relationships. Yet we take loving action for granted or stop short at simply being nice to people, which is not enough. How often do we consciously take time to love on someone when they are down, or even when we are down? It's much easier to let the emotion pass or go to the gym or a bar. Be honest with yourself: Could you take a little extra time to help someone, to volunteer for an hour, to consciously express gratitude for the things you have in your life? I could. We all could, and should, especially since it will not only benefit someone else but our own health as well.

When you love someone, go deep. Use your logical brain to tune into their emotions. Try to fundamentally and impactfully improve their life. Think about all the benefits associated with living a life of love. How great does it feel when you give selflessly and effortlessly to someone in need? When you commit to accomplishing something and persist through the tough times until it is finished? When you uniquely express yourself to someone and they return the gesture with love and compassion?

Love is an action, an act of free will. Yes, love is associated with positive emotions, but *to love* is to do things for other people. To be selfless. To sacrifice for a greater purpose. To act with the expectation of nothing in return.

Love is and always will be the goal, the objective, the solution, the reason, the answer to *anything* in life: why we are here, where we came from, what we are to do, where we are going, how we can better ourselves and others. Love is willing the good of another. Goodness is directing something toward its ultimate purpose. In our case, it is exercising divine attributes—intelligence, logic, virtue, creativity, communication—which produces beauty and reveals truth. Truth means (in my humble opinion) that we are made in the image of God and that our ultimate purpose is to love, which improves our well-being and gives meaning to our lives.

Part 3: Practice – Stress Reduction

Breaking Bad Habits

Remember, it is the automatic, unconscious, nonrational parts of our brain that drive both our habitual stress response and our coping mechanisms. We need to take conscious action to break those unhealthy habits and develop new habitual thoughts and actions. Ideally, we'll also find meaning and purpose and manifest greater love, so that we can live more fulfilled lives. All will improve our well-being.

These activities have been scientifically shown to improve brain function and promote ease in the mind and body. The idea is to practice them consistently—some daily—so that over time, you won't have to push yourself to do them. You'll either want to do them or they will have become unconscious habits.

We are creatures of habit because the brain runs on autopilot most of the time. From an ancient-ancestral perspective, repetition and familiarity helped keep us safe. In *The Power of Habit: Why We Do What We Do in Life and Business*, journalist Charles Duhigg describes three components to habits, which he calls the habit loop. The *cue* is what triggers the habit. The *routine* is the action that occurs in response to the cue. The *reward* is the feeling or emotion that results from the action.[1] Here's an example of the habit loop involving stress:

The cue = stress

The routine = consuming sugar-filled foods

The reward = the release of dopamine, a feel-good chemical in the brain

The result = sugar cravings, obesity, diabetes, and other health problems

To eliminate a bad habit that has resulted from stress, we need to eliminate the cue. Since the stress itself may be habitual, it's important to understand where it is coming from. In my case, changing a habit developed in response to my stress—my cookie bingeing—helped me focus on dealing with the source of my stress.

B.J. Fogg, PhD, a computer scientist who founded and directs research and design at the Stanford Behavior Design Lab, at Stanford University, has concluded that the way to break bad habits is to start small, with what he calls tiny habits. Break the habit into its component parts (cue, routine, reward), focus on your behavior (the routine), and add a simple new behavior to immediately follow it. It should be something easy to do, so that regardless of willpower, it will likely get done, which takes motivation out of the equation.[2]

Let's use my stress and sweets as an example. If I place the package of Oreos next to a bowl of fruit, that will force me to at least look at the fruit the next time I reach for the cookies. I may not eat any the first time, or the second or third time, but eventually I will. And that is a big win, which I should be proud of. According to Dr. Fogg, I should give myself a pat on the back or raise my hands in the air and shout "Awesome!"

In fact, each time you choose the healthy behavior over the

unhealthy habit, reward yourself emotionally: smiling, pumping your arms in victory, telling yourself, "Nice job, woo hoo! I feel great!" Might sounds silly, but it works!

I found that you can literally change the way you feel by carrying yourself in a confident, powerful manner. And good posture is one of the easiest habits to develop. As you go about your day, stand up tall, lift your chin up, stick your chest out slightly, and smile. Walk a little faster, with a bit of a spring in your step. Loosen your muscles. Look people in the eye.

The most powerful, longest-lasting rewards are emotional in nature. And small steps can lead to large outcomes.

Keystone Habits

Charles Duhigg says that we can create the biggest change in our lifestyle by adopting a habit that will lead to other new habits, and multiple new behaviors. He calls this a keystone habit. Meditation is my keystone habit.

The early-morning hours, before the hustle and bustle of the day, are a good time to work on the mind. At first, it was hard to wake up at five a.m., but once I started reaping the benefits, it became easier and easier.

I noticed that what I ate for dinner the night before had an effect on my energy the next day. The better my diet, the easier it was to wake up, so I started eating healthier throughout the day, too. Eventually, I didn't need to set my alarm; my body had become conditioned to waking up at five a.m. exactly. And I was excited to get out of bed, to meditate and perform activities that were harder to fit into my schedule, like reading, journaling, and exercising.

Because of my morning routine, I was able to get a lot of things done before my workday began. I was happier at work, with better focus and concentration. I smiled at people and interacted more. I was better at controlling my emotions. I had more energy. I came home and engaged with my wife and kids more. All because I developed a keystone habit of meditation.

Meditation

When we are feeling relaxed and contemplative, our brain waves slow into alpha and theta states, and the unconscious regions of the brain become highly active. Hypnotherapists guide their patients into the theta state so that they can become more suggestible. The slower the brain-wave state, the deeper into the unconscious we go.

Our brains operate in alpha/theta states just before we fall asleep and just before we wake up. That's why early in the morning and just before going to sleep, when the mind has had a chance to calm down, are excellent times to meditate.[3] Of course, meditation can be practiced at any time. Ideally, you want to find a place with minimal sound (complete silence is helpful but not necessary) and no interruptions: on the couch in the morning, in bed at night, in a quiet room at the office, in your car in a quiet parking lot.

As little as 10 minutes a day can provide a benefit. Even five minutes at first is a win. Then try for 10 minutes, then 20, and then 30.... however long it takes to hit that deep relaxing sensation that changes the way you're feeling physically and mentally.

The first time you try it, there's a good chance you'll only feel a little more relaxed. That calm feeling of relaxation is great itself! If you are anything like I was, with my brain going full blast for years, it's going to take some time to take control of it and step outside of it. But once that occurs, your stress levels will begin to plummet.

Here's a simple meditation practice I use daily: Sit quietly in a comfortable position, spine erect, eyes closed, and just focus on your breathing. Concentrate on breathing in and out through your nose; listen to your breathing sounds; feel your belly moving in and out as you inhale and exhale.

If you hear something that generates a thought or a thought pops into your head, let it occur and then let it go. Acknowledge your thoughts without judgment, notice them coming and going, and bring your conscious awareness back to your breathing. If your mind starts paying attention to something in your environment, like the surface you're sitting on, that's fine, too. Recognize it, feel it, and then bring your focus back to your breathing. Pulling your attention back to your breath is like doing pullups for your brain.

By closing your eyes and putting yourself in this position, you have essentially turned off four of the five senses. This is an integral part of the meditative process. After a few minutes, you should start to lose sensation in your arms and legs and then, depending on how long your session lasts, in the rest of your body. This is perfectly normal and good! You'll be aware of feelings of tranquility, peace, selflessness, even being out-of-body, in a sense. Your mind will be fully alert and yet your body will be completely relaxed—just the opposite of a stress response. It's that simple.

After you practice this meditation a few times, you will find it easier to enter into the relaxed state, quiet your mind, focus your attention, and consciously direct your thoughts.

Here are two other forms of meditation that I find extremely helpful—and, with respect to the content of this book, fitting:

Loving-kindness meditation: Focus your thoughts on love—love toward yourself, love toward another person, love toward a higher power. Imagine yourself full of perfect love and directing that love toward someone in your life. Concentrate on bringing that love into that life through your words and actions, and the love that person will feel in return. Focus on the love you have for yourself in that moment. Relive a loving experience you have had with a loved one, a companion or friend, a child. Focus on the perfect love you are receiving in that moment from your creator.

Gratitude meditation: Focus on the beautiful gift of life you feel with every breath and heartbeat. Give thanks for this very moment, your beating heart, the safety and comfort of your surroundings. Give thanks for your family, your friends, the opportunity to use your unique mind and abilities to better the lives of others. Give thanks for the things you have and the things you want to bring into your life. Give thanks to yourself for working to improve your life so that you can improve the lives of others. Give thanks for the relaxing sensation of meditation.

Mindfulness

Mindfulness is a simple technique that can be incorporated into a meditative session. Beyond that, you can practice it at any time in any situation: at work, in the car, during a family gathering. It involves consciously focusing on your thoughts and feelings and the sensations around you; on what is occurring right here and now, not what happened in the past or might happen in the future.

Once you finish this paragraph, pause for a moment. Pay attention to your heart rate, your breathing, the clothes touching your skin, the thoughts running through your head, what you hear, what you see in front of you. Do not analyze or judge; just observe dispassionately. Do this for a few seconds. You are being mindful.

When you pay this kind of attention to whatever you're doing—focusing solely on the task at hand, using all your senses to take in every detail—even simple activities like washing the dishes or cutting the grass can become more enjoyable.

When you eat, chew your food slowly and savor each bite. Pay attention to the sensation and taste of each mouthful. Being more aware of your brain's signals means you'll note when you've had enough, which should prevent overeating and a mindless reach for more. In my case, the more fulfillment I derived from transcendent sources and contributive actions, the less interested I was in eating as a source of enjoyment.

When you exercise, feel the strain and tension in the individual muscles. Let's use biceps curls as an example. Focus on the upward movement as you curl the dumbbell toward your shoulder; on the downward motion as you return it to your hip. As you watch yourself in the mirror, concentrate on perfect form. Feel pride in your work and your workout, knowing how they are improving your body and health.

Mindfulness and yoga go hand in hand. While you are holding a pose, focus your attention on controlling your breathing. Direct your thoughts to your body and feel the release of tension as you transition from move to move, breathing out stress and anxiety. This will help put you into a calm, Zen-like state that benefits the brain as you physically challenge your body.

Be mindful of the cue in the habit loop. Think about what causes the unhealthy behavior you want to change. Recognize the trigger. Pay close attention to your behavior and, instead of thinking about the reward, focus on the negative aspects of what you're doing. If you eat too many sweets, recognize that consuming so much sugar can lead to brain fog, an upset stomach, cavities, even diabetes; that a sugar crash can leave you tired and perhaps feeling worse than before. Focusing on these downsides can outweigh the short-term dopamine reward and make it easier to avoid or start cutting down on sweets.

Conversely, take the time after any health-improving activity to concentrate on the good feelings it generated: calmness after meditating, energy after a workout, compassion after a charity event. That feeling helps to encode a powerful memory that you can draw upon in the future.

Mindfulness and Time

Mindfulness—you can also call it *awareness*—is the first step in making any kind of change as it pertains to stress and health. We have to observe exactly what it is that is stressing us out, what we are doing to cope with the stress, and how our bodies and minds are reacting.

Many times, it is time itself that is causing us stress. Often, we don't know how to manage it properly. We are always rushing to the next task; we waste time on activities we think we should be doing or "have to" get done. We waste more time on things we believe will bring us happiness, like going to the bar for a few drinks, and sacrifice being present in the moment. Before we know it, years have gone by and we're asking ourselves, "Where did my life go?"

As we get older, time can be a huge source of anxiety as we feel it moving faster and faster. There's a reason for that. When we are young, each day seems different—because in many ways it is. We are learning so much, having so many different experiences, feeling so many vibrant emotions that essentially anchor those events in our brains, forming strong memories. We live more in the moment and pay more attention to details.

And the older we get, the more common it is to come across information we already know. Since the brain is always looking for shortcuts, it tends not to reprocess this information and moves on to the next task or thought. No wonder we are forming less detailed memories. We rarely stop to enjoy the moment, soak in all its vivid aspects, tap into our emotional state.

But if we do—that is, if we take time each day to take note of that moment, using all our senses to create detailed mental pictures, which turn into memories—we can slow our perception of time and eliminate it as a source of stress. I know when I really pay attention to something, the clock seems to move more slowly. The same goes for when I meditate. It is when I am all scatterbrained and distracted that the time flies by.

Interoception

The body is constantly sending signals to the brain. Interoception is a specific form of mindfulness by which we tune in to physiological details. When you notice how stressful situations affect, for instance, your heart rate, perspiration, body temperature, and muscle tightness, you can move more quickly to eliminate the stress.[4]

This doesn't apply only to stress, of course. If you practice interoception while working out, you can better sense how hard to push during a workout, when to increase or decrease force or repetition, and when you need to take a break.

According to a 2015 article in *Psychology Today*, "the correlation between interoceptive awareness and emotion has become increasingly well established." The article looked at a study published in *NeuroImage* in 2012, in which the subjects monitored their heartbeats as they watched videos of people telling emotion-filled stories. Each time, the subjects showed "similar patterns of activation in the insular cortex—the region deep inside the brain responsible for both emotional feelings and interoception." This supported the idea, the researchers wrote, that awareness of our bodies and our emotions are "intimately linked."

The article also noted that low interoceptive awareness has been associated with "depersonalization disorder," eating disorders, depression, and unexplained physical symptoms, such as pain.[5]

Interestingly, at least one study has shown that people who pay attention to their heartbeats are more giving than those who do not. The researchers attempted to gauge if the "participants' sensitivity to their own heartbeat" could predict their decision in several situations in which they were asked to choose between self-interest and altruism. The study, published in *Scientific Reports* in 2017, found that "People with higher interoceptive sensitivity are more altruistic."[6] This is why it's important to listen to your heart!

The study found that improving interoception skills did not increase altruism, although I like to think it just takes practice. Listen to your body and feel the biological sensations when you're performing any health-related activities, from meditation and mindfulness to exercise and eating. When you are exercising, feel your heart rate and respiratory rate; notice your body temperature and levels of perspiration. When you are eating, pay attention to how full your stomach is as compared to your feeling of satiation. When you are in a stress response, note the tension in your body, your pounding heart, your heavier breathing.

Once you are aware of what your emotional and survival brains are causing you to do, you can use your logical brain to calm yourself with rational thoughts: "This is just your body reacting normally to a perceived threat" or "You are fine, this will pass in two minutes." Don't forget to start breathing slowly and deeply.

Visualization

Also referred to as mental imagery or mental rehearsal, visualization is the act of constructing vivid pictures of situations or actions in your mind and imagining you are living in that moment, like Michael Phelps did with swimming. Envision hitting that perfect golf shot, nailing a job presentation or a musical performance, crossing the finish line of your first marathon. Create every little detail, as well as potential obstacles, and your brain will be much better equipped to tackle those situations. Creating such images in the mind is just as important as practicing physically. And practicing often is critical.

Often, when I felt stressed or fearful, I would relive and replay all the sights, sounds, and emotions of one of the greatest days of my life: my wedding day. I would put myself back at the reception and on the dance floor. I would feel the passionate love for my new bride, the joy of seeing all my relatives in one place (which doesn't happen often); I would hear the incredible band we'd hired, see the beautiful lighting and flower arrangements; feel myself energetically dancing and singing with my wife and friends. After a few moments, I would feel as if I were literally there on that joyous day.

Now you try: Imagine one of the happiest events in *your* life—your wedding, the birth of a child, a holiday gathering with family, an exciting accomplishment at work. Create a mental image of that event as if you were experiencing it today, extremely bright and detailed, with vibrant color, sound, smell, touch. See the smiles on the faces of your loved ones; hear the praise of your colleagues; touch the tears of happiness on your face; taste the celebratory champagne. Feel the warm sensation of pure love and joy throughout your body, driving you to share that energy with the outside world.

Gerald Epstein, M.D., a psychiatrist, has used visualization techniques in his practice for decades. A book he co-edited, *The Encyclopedia of Mental Imagery: Colette Aboulker-Muscat's 2,100 Visualizations for Personal Development, Healing and Self-Knowledge*, which describes an array of mental-imagery exercises he uses with his patients, is a good reference.[7]

Affirmation

If visualization is "seeing," affirmation (some use the term *self-affirmation*) is "speaking"—that is, talking to yourself. The act of communicating with yourself has also been shown to help regulate emotions and increase a sense of self-worth, particularly when contemplating future scenarios.[8]

Three experiments described in the *European Journal of Social Psychology* in 2014 and reprinted in the Wiley Online Library suggest that talking to yourself in the second person—using *you* rather than the first-person *I*—strengthens both behavior and intentions. That's what I do during affirming moments. Talking to myself is another activity that seemed strange at first but was surprisingly helpful in overcoming my negative emotions.[9]

Say I found myself stressing over a phone call from a customer, asking for help when I was already swamped. I would mentally yell at myself as if I were one of my football coaches. "Are you kidding me? She just needs help looking up data on a patient! Is that so hard? It will take one minute! It's your job! And she doesn't know how busy you are, so why are you getting so angry? C'mon, calm down! Take a deep breath, put on a smile, and go make someone's day a little easier."

Aggressive talk in my athletic career helped me perform better—funny how this time it was all about empathy and willing the good of another. I wouldn't use this approach for every situation, and I'm not necessarily advocating it, but it worked for me, because sometimes I need a kick in the butt.

I also use affirmation during visualization sessions. For instance, when I envision giving a speech to my colleagues, I always sprinkle in a little encouragement: "You've got this!" "You are going to be great!" "You know you're well prepared, so go out there and have fun!"

It's important to think about how you phrase something. If you're feeling relaxed, don't say, "You are full of energy and on fire today!" because your body is not reflecting that state. If you tell yourself, "This is a small problem," the brain might ignore all the words except the negative word *problem*. Simply saying words without the appropriate emotion can also backfire and even cause more stress and fear, if the affirmations are not believable.

During meditation or visualization sessions to strengthen neural pathways and focus on positive energy, utter phrases in your head like "You are in control" or "You are calm and at peace" or "You are full of love." When you envision a scenario such as having a difficult conversation with a loved one, remind yourself, "You can do this" or "Everything will be fine, because you want the best outcome and are doing this out of love."

If you feel yourself slipping back into old habits or becoming stressed out, tell yourself, "Don't worry, you can handle this" or "You can calm yourself down." Then reinforce the statement with a postural change or breathing technique.

Stand Tall and Breathe
As I said earlier, one of the first things I did to calm my stress and fear was to stand with my chin up, shoulders back, and chest out slightly. You can change the way you feel just by carrying yourself in a more confident, powerful manner.

And simple breathing techniques can help stop the stress response dead in its tracks. An easy way to incorporate them in your life is to start and end your day with a few minutes of controlled breathing. Here are a few breathing techniques that promote relaxation. Perform these exercises until you feel calm or relaxed:

Deep controlled breathing: Inhale through the nose for four seconds; exhale through the mouth (or nose) for eight seconds.

Alternate-nostril breathing: Close your right nostril, inhale through the left nostril, and hold your breath for three seconds. Then close your left nostril, exhale through the right one, and hold your breath for three seconds. This time inhale through your right nostril as your left one is closed, and repeat the technique, alternating nostrils.

Diaphragmatic breathing: Lie down, stretch out, put your hands on your abdomen, and concentrate on taking slow, deep breaths, in through the nose and out through the mouth (or breathing in and out of your nose, if you prefer). Feel your abdomen expand and contract. Visualize your lungs full of air after each inhalation and completely empty after each exhalation. Don't worry about how long you inhale or exhale; let it occur naturally.

Progressive Muscle Relaxation

A related exercise is progressive muscle relaxation, or PMR, the simple practice of tightening one muscle group at a time, then releasing that tension and relaxing. You can do this seated or lying down. Typically, you'd start with the lower extremities—feet, ankles, and leg—and end with your shoulders, neck, and head.

I found that when combined with deep breathing, PMR helped me fall asleep more quickly. So many nights, after reliving the day's events in my head, I'd get upset thinking about the next day. Who wouldn't? But when I directed my thoughts to individual body parts, one by one, my body relaxed, which helped relax my mind. That made it easier to focus on my breath work, and that really made it easier to fall asleep.

An article on the website WebMD, "Progressive Muscle Relaxation Technique for Stress and Insomnia," notes that doctors have used PMR with standard treatments for the relief of symptoms associated with headaches, cancer pain, high blood pressure, and digestive disturbances.[10] Here are their instructions:

1. While breathing in, contract your lower left leg (foot and calf) for five to ten seconds, then suddenly relax those muscles as you breathe out. As you do that, you might visualize the stressful feelings flowing out of your body.
2. Focus on the relaxation sensation you feel in your lower leg.
3. Rest for ten to twenty seconds, then move on to your left thigh.
4. Repeat with your right foot, calf, and thigh.
5. Move on to your abdomen and chest and repeat these steps.
6. Repeat with your left hand and arm and then your right.
7. Finish with your shoulders, neck, and head.

Cognitive Restructuring

Cognitive restructuring has to do with analyzing negative thinking and asking questions that will lead to new conclusions. It is rooted in the Socratic method: pointed questioning intended to challenge ideas with logical thinking. The process involves becoming aware of your negative thinking, challenging those thoughts by modifying the rationale given them, and employing better logic.

Here are some examples of Socratic questioning used in cognitive restructuring:[11]

* Are these feelings or facts?
* Are these thoughts just assumptions?
* Could my thinking be an exaggeration of the truth?
* Is there an alternative explanation?
* What evidence do I have to verify my opinion?

* Am I looking at all the evidence?

* What are the best-case and worst-case outcomes? How likely are they?

* Is my thought a likely scenario or a worst-case outcome?

I used to worry about a wide variety of things, from losing my job to giving a ten-minute presentation in a work meeting. My questions were not Socratic but simply stress inducing: "What if I forget what I plan to say? I always get nervous when speaking in public; what is everyone going to think of me if I stutter? Why does my manager keep asking me to make these presentations? I'm not even good at it."

If I let them persist, these thoughts would make me feel embarrassed and ashamed. And frankly, they were a distortion of the truth about my skills. Thankfully, after my meditation and mindfulness training, I was able to recognize and head off these thoughts. Then I would use the cognitive-reframing technique and challenge them with some Socratic questioning:

Are these thoughts just assumptions? Yes. Even though I get a little nervous before speaking in front of people, that is perfectly normal, and people often say how relaxed and confident I seem.

Is there any evidence for these thoughts? No. My manager often tells me he asks me to convey new information to my peers because I do a good job.

Do these thoughts describe a likely scenario? No. I always prepare for my presentations, and my nervousness evaporates once I get started.

Is there an alternate explanation for this negative thinking? Yes. It is just my brain's way of helping me avoid things that are out of my comfort zone or a little scary. Remember, the brain can't tell the difference between a presentation and a hungry tiger; any fear triggers the survival mode.

With cognitive restructuring, we can challenge our unhealthy thinking with logic, view our situations and ourselves in a more reasonable light, and replace negative thoughts and emotions with positive ones. Once I reasoned through my negative thoughts in this way, my mindset changed, and the fear dissipated.

Journaling

Writing down your thoughts consolidates your memories and adds clarity to your thinking.[12] Because of the deeper thinking and cognitive complexity associated with writing, it is heavily used in cognitive behavioral therapy. I found it really helps to change the way I think, feel, and act.

Journaling is what led me to write this book! As I researched the best ways to manage stress, I came across so much powerful information that sparked my thinking that I felt compelled to write it down. The practices I read about and started adopting changed my brain and body, so I wrote about how that made me feel. I wrote about my negative emotions and stress, what was causing those feelings, and how I could use certain techniques to better manage them.

As I read the work of great philosophers like Socrates,

Aristotle, and Anselm, I would take their thoughts and apply them to my life. I analyzed my place in the universe and my views on the world. Journaling really got the wheels turning, especially regarding my new philosophical thinking about life, meaning, and purpose. I often had random thoughts that I wanted to capture, so I would dictate a note on my phone and later add it to my journal.

Eventually, my journal grew into hundreds of pages. The process of describing and analyzing my thoughts and feelings helped me develop a strategy to improve my well-being, and once that happened, I took everything I had and put it into this book.

Revisiting a journal generates self-awareness. Reflecting on what you've written facilitates new thoughts. For example, when journaling about something that gives you anxiety, like the amount of work you have to do at your job each day, you can analyze the situation, develop a plan on how to address it, and start to rectify it. You might create a to-do list for the day, adding how soon each item needs to be done, who could help you with it, what you might say to your manager in asking for help, and your goal for finishing everything. Once you've completed all the tasks, you might list everything that would improve your workload going forward.

Think about exactly what you want to accomplish. Buy a notebook and write in it every day. Describe your feelings and express yourself honestly. Create a mantra that you will read and recite each day. Construct a vision and plan for health or other improvements, set goals, and take action! Look for ways to bring your thoughts and goals to life each day, then write about it in your journal. If you learn something from reading or talking to someone, from watching a video or listening to a podcast, write about that, too.

Accountability

There should be no doubt (certainly, I hope, after you've gone through this book!) that people can change their brains. Managing stress and negative emotions, strengthening beliefs, forming new healthy habits—these are key to living life to the fullest. You don't need anyone else to do it. You don't need any gadgets, tracking devices, motivational videos or apps. You are all you need to change.

That said, you've spent years developing habits, beliefs, and actions that can be challenging to alter. Other people can help you get started and coach you along the way. Plus, it's more fun and often easier to go at it with another person or a group of people.

An article in *Psychology Today* in 2016 described some experiments into this phenomenon, known as the Social Facilitation Effect, at Stanford two years earlier. In one experiment, the researchers told subjects who were working on a puzzle alone that others were working on the puzzle as well. With a second group, there was no mention of working with anyone else.

Tips on how to complete the puzzle were presented to both groups. The first group received memos with a "To" line and a "From" line, implying that they came from someone working on the puzzle (and not from the person leading the experiment). The second group received memos that had only a "For" line and the participant's name. Those in the first group described working on the puzzle as more enjoyable, worked longer and performed better, and were more likely to choose to come back for a related task than those in the second group.

In an earlier experiment cited in the same article, participants who were jogging with someone who supposedly had the same birthday increased their heart rate as the other person's heart rate increased and reported feeling more connected to the other jogger than those who were not told about matching birthdays.[13]

It can be very tough to hold ourselves accountable to new actions, especially health-related ones, if we've never done them before and don't see immediate results. That is normal, because our brains have spent years seeking shortcuts to conserve energy and bring us pleasure, even if they're bad for our long-term health.

When I first started my morning routine, I asked my brother to do it with me. The notion came at just the right time for my brother, who was getting out of a highly dysfunctional relationship and was using unhealthy coping mechanisms. (In fact, many of the articles I was researching were just as much for him as for me.) We would set our alarms for five a.m. and text or call each other to make sure we were awake.

Sometimes we would spend a little time talking about our lives and health, or life itself. For me, our conversations often led to a journal entry or a hard workout. It didn't take long before I was able to wake up on my own, but having him there in the beginning was a huge help.

If we could only exercise self-control, we wouldn't need an

accountability partner. But self-control is what we are trying to develop! We tend to tell ourselves, "I want a healthy mind and body, but there's no way I can get up early to meditate!" Or "I want to eat better and lose weight, but it is going to take such hard work, and the workouts may be painful."

I know how hard it is to fight the urge for that cookie, especially when eating it isn't going to hurt me right now. It's easier to say, "I'll start jogging tomorrow" than to lace up my shoes and get out the door. Our brains drive us down the easy, more familiar path. To overcome that unhealthy tendency, we need to get creative about gaining a reward in the here and now.

Here's where an accountability partner can be so helpful. You can accomplish anything you need to do on your own. But, especially in the beginning, it's a great idea to find a coach, mentor or partner, or join a group to provide you with education, feedback, and support. It's also much more fulfilling to experience positive change with other people. Sharing the journey with others helps facilitate positive change in their lives as well!

Thinking

Take a long look at your reality—your loved ones, your job, your friends, every aspect of your life—and go deep. What is causing your stress and why? Keep asking "Why?" until you can go no further.

For example, your job is stressing you out. Why? Because my manager is always asking me to do more, and I don't have enough time. Why can't you make time? Because I have a wife and three kids, and my plate is full. It's hard enough to maintain focus and productivity at work. Why? Because I'm always so tired. What can you do to improve your sleep? And so on. Get the idea?

Then go deeper. Learn and think about whatever interests you, whether science, philosophy, art or literature, something that pertains to your job or a hobby. Use that knowledge to improve your situation.

Throughout my health-improvement journey, I was constantly filling my mind with new and thought-provoking information. In the morning, I read countless books on science, philosophy, health and well-being. Driving to and from work and from one hospital to the next, I listened to numerous audiobooks and podcasts, often more than once. I captured hundreds of pages of thoughts in my journal and conveyed what I learned to family and friends.

Whenever I came across a deep philosophical principle, I would meditate on it, think about the truth of the matter, even record myself talking about it. I loved diving into those big life questions! By doing so, I gained clarity and direction. And I felt compelled to share everything, which helped me learn the material better. Remember: Neurons that fire together, wire together. It's all about repetition.

Daily conscious thoughts pertaining to meaning, purpose, love, relationships, logic, philosophy, beauty, truth, and goodness lead to greater health and well-being. Thoughts lead to actions and subsequent healthy emotion, and as a result, new beliefs are formed. Flood your brain and mind with uplifting, thought-provoking content; meditate daily; take action that generates positive, loving emotion, which reinforces these deeper thoughts and beliefs.

In the beginning, it may take a great amount of conscious effort. The key is to focus not on your emotions but on rationality and critical thinking. Use your logical brain to take action because you know it will be beneficial; the results may not come immediately but they *will* come. Don't wait until you "feel like" making a change. *Act as you should, not as you feel.* Take charge of your stress now.

Taking control of your conscious awareness—practicing mindfulness—can affect unconscious processes and unconscious, habitual feelings and manifestations of beliefs. Be more conscious. Be more philosophical. Go deeper with your thoughts, feelings, and actions. Practice meditation, affirmations, and visualization in the morning and be mindful the rest of the day.

Yes, your mind will wander, but bring yourself back to the present, whether you are engaged in a task or with a person. Use all your senses to take in each precious moment. This will help you form strong, vivid memories and can also slow down your perception of time. There is no time like the present.

We have incredible logical and rational capabilities. Why not tackle the big questions? Why not pursue knowledge of the source of life? Why not use divine empathy and strive for perfection?

Don't just be nice to somebody; be empathetic and will the good of another, *any* other, at any and all times. Do something to make their day and life a bit better. In this way, encourage them to do the same for other people.

Express yourself in the most beautiful ways to the highest degree possible. Contemplate life's meaning and purpose and take action every day toward realizing them. Not only will your health and well-being improve; so will your relationships and your impact on the lives of others.

Daily Routine

Here's an example of my morning routine and what I do the rest of the day. The times, durations, and order of actions are not important. Sometimes I exercise, sometimes I read, sometimes I meditate or write for longer than I did the morning before. The key is to include reading, meditation, and journaling every morning.

5:00 a.m. – Wake up
5:15 a.m. – Reading
5:30 a.m. – Journaling
5:45 a.m. – Breathing and meditation, visualization, affirmation
6:00 a.m. – Exercise
2:00 p.m. – Breathing, meditation, thinking, cognitive restructuring
9:00 p.m. – TEE time (thought, emotion, experience) with my wife
9:30 p.m. – Breathing, PMR, gratitude or loving meditation
10:00 p.m.– Go to sleep

At first, I simply read a little, wrote a little, and meditated for a few minutes each morning. I also meditated mid-day.

After I got used to waking up early and began seeing the benefits of these actions, I added visualization, affirmation, and exercise in the form of running, biking, or weightlifting. I used my breathing techniques and postural changes in times of stress and exercised when I had the opportunity. Actually, a little bit of good stress each day, like exercise, is beneficial to health and promotes neuroplasticity.[14] Combined with the meditation, those activities really helped me recharge my mind and body.

Most important, my routine gave me control over my conscious thinking. Eventually, I found myself doing more for the people I interacted with. Instead of getting frustrated from repetitive calls from a customer, I picked up the phone and offered immediate help. Instead of just taking care of the problem and hanging up, I conversed for a few minutes. I could hear the person's tone of voice change and pictured the smile on the other end of the line.

I tried putting more smiles on more faces throughout the day. It is such a simple concept, but something I had overlooked for years. I had had every opportunity to feel more fulfilled, both at work and at home; it was simply up to me to take action to make it happen.

We *can* reduce our stress, change our brains and our minds, and realize greater meaning and purpose in life. Let my routine help you create a routine for yourself, filled with practices I've described here. Then find an accountability partner to help you develop a habit of consistent action. Don't stop until you see results, because they will come!

These practices and ways of thinking helped me in so many ways. I know, if you put in the time and effort, they will help you, too.

Appendix - God and Health

I am often asked about my belief in God and how it is linked to health, happiness, and a sense of purpose in life. Clearly, we don't have to believe in a higher power to live healthy lives full of love and goodness. The actions outlined in this book (and indeed, in many other health and wellness programs) draw from ancient and modern spiritual practices that exist across nearly all traditions. If a higher power exists and we are acting with love and goodness, we are tapping into that higher power whether we choose to believe so or not.

But I believe our physical reality can't provide the highest degree of health, fulfillment, or purpose. If God exists, that means there is a nonphysical aspect to our existence that is the ultimate source of our health and well-being. And we can connect to God through our minds. We can access God through logical thought.

An Argument for the Existence and Nature of God

All my reading in philosophy over the years led naturally to books on metaphysics. Once I started asking those big questions—why are we here, where did we come from, what are we supposed to do, where are we going—I wound up at the biggest ones: Does God exist? If so, what is God like? What does that mean for my life? I discovered answers that so profoundly affected my worldview and well-being, I want to share them here.

I agree with Edward Feser, PhD, a professor of philosophy at Pasadena City College, in California. In his book *Five Proofs of the*

Existence of God, he examines the thinking of some of the greatest philosophers in history and their conclusions that the existence of God can be established by way of purely rational thinking.[1] This notion is a little deep, but well worth diving into.

Everything that we observe in the world is moving and changing. Change entails going from *potential* to *actual*. For example, if I am standing on a green over a golf ball, the ball is *potentially* in the cup. If I putt well, it moves forward and is soon *actually* in the cup. You can say its potential has been actualized.

My point is that in any situation involving change, something *actual* must exist to cause that change. Something had to cause the ball to move from potentially dropping into the cup to resting on the bottom. In this case, the golf club was that cause, but its action, too, was only potential until I actualized it. Just as the ball possessed only the potential to drop into the cup until the golf club hit it in, the club possessed only the potential to hit the ball until I took it out of my bag and used it.

We could continue running this thought exercise deeper and deeper: I had the potential to swing the club until doing so was actualized by my arms, whose movement was actualized by my brain, whose ability to work is actualized by cells, atoms, and subatomic particles.

Eventually, we have to reach a fundamental point and source of pure actuality—that is, something that itself has no potential and needs no actualizing. This entity is not contingent upon anything else to move it or change it, or for its existence. This entity must exist, because if it didn't, we would have an infinite regress of causes and effects, with no ultimate first cause. I think that would be logically and philosophically absurd.

If there were no such entity, there would be no ultimate explanation of the changes we see here and now in our everyday lives. Everything in our reality is dependent upon something already actual beyond itself to move or change. Nothing actualizes itself.

Change is occurring at all times, in every circumstance, in every place in the universe. *Something* has to be causing all this movement, something that itself is changeless—nothing is required to actualize it. It actualizes all potentials and yet is purely actual itself. It is thus a changeless entity, an "unmoved mover," as Aristotle put it thousands of years ago, the prime mover.[2] That would make it the foundation for all reality and all existence.

If an uncaused entity that transcends our reality exists, there are significant implications. If this entity has no potential, then it can't exist in time and space, because everything in time and space undergoes change. It can't consist of energy or matter, because energy and matter undergo change. It must be infinite, because if it were finite, it would at some point cease to exist, which means that it would change. It couldn't have just popped into existence at some point because that, too, would indicate change.

Furthermore, in order to create, move, and change everything, this entity must have maximum power. Perfect intellect, perfect goodness, love, beauty, and every other beneficial feature of reality must also be part of its nature. If not, it would have only the potential for these maximum attributes; it couldn't be purely actual.

So, what is this fundamental primary cause? Since everything within our realm of understanding undergoes change, even subatomic particles and energy lack the perfect, maximum, infinite characteristics of an "unmoved mover." On the other hand, what many people refer to as God is a very reasonable candidate. Not the old, bearded, judgmental man in the sky, but rather a perfectly loving, perfectly good, nonphysical source of existence that is creating and sustaining life at this very moment.

From this line of Aristotelian thinking (and plenty of other influences that I've left out), my confidence in the truth of reality skyrocketed, as did my ability to process stress and hardship. As I've said before, my stress came mostly from fearful thinking. When I set my thoughts on purpose and meaning, and took virtuous action stemming from those thoughts, my fear and stress diminished dramatically.

Free Will and Leibniz Optimism

Now, I know what you may be thinking; I wondered the same thing for a long time. If the source of all reality is perfect love and perfect goodness, why is there so much pain and suffering in the world? If God exists, how can evil, the utter absence of goodness and love, also exist? The answer, I believe, lies in the notion of free will.

We humans have used our free will since the birth of the species to perform brutal actions, to inflict harm on one another, to alter the environment in ways that cause sickness and disease.

Freedom is very good, and perfect love entails willing the good of every human being equally. It follows that since God allows all humans to make free choices, God would not stop the evil in the world.

Emotionally, I find this very hard to accept. Anyone would, especially those who have suffered at the hands of another. But from a logical perspective, I believe it makes sense. Doing evil is a choice that humans freely make, and stopping them would mean robbing them of their free will.

Once I accepted that the existence of evil and of God were not incompatible, I began to wonder about existence itself. The world did not have to be the way it is—we could have lived in some other kind of world—yet if God exists, and if God created the world, the world must be the way it is supposed to be. I take great comfort in the notions of Gottfried Wilhelm Leibniz, a scientist and philosopher and one of the great thinkers of the seventeenth and eighteenth centuries. Among his philosophical principles, in what is now referred to as Leibniz Optimism, he argues that the world we find ourselves in is the best possible world we could, in principle, live in.[3]

But how can that be? How can this be the *best* possible world? Because God's nature includes perfect intelligence and power, it follows that any kind of world could have been created, Leibniz argued, or no world at all. Because God is all-knowing and all-powerful, though, God knew which world was best and was able to create it. Since God's nature is also that of perfect love and goodness, it follows that God created the best of all possible worlds out of love.

Craig's Philosophy

But if God exists, why make belief so difficult? Again, using a little rational thought, we can come up with some compelling reasons. Perhaps God intended to provide just the right amount of evidence for humans to exercise a little hope, faith, critical thinking, curiosity, and wonder with respect to God's existence. Maybe if God were present in a much greater capacity or we were certain that God existed, we would have a lesser degree of faith, less curiosity to seek God out.

Or maybe we would essentially turn into robots, worshipping God in a manner that robbed us of free will. In fact, if we had absolute certainty of God's existence and, say, lost a loved one too soon, we might even turn against God in our grief or anger.

William Lane Craig, a research professor in philosophy at the Talbot School of Theology at Biola University, near Los Angeles, a philosophy professor at Houston Baptist University, and the author of *God Over All*, suggests that if God placed a neon symbol among the stars, more people might believe, but people might also "chafe under the brazen advertisements of their creator and even come to resent such effrontery."[4] It makes sense that God would desire a loving relationship with us, and a scenario in which God is "more present" could have the opposite effect or prevent the return of love given freely.

Perhaps God isn't absent, however, but completely accessible at any time through human reasoning. Since God is love and goodness, when we set our thoughts on love and goodness and take actions that reflect this, we are inevitably connecting with God. I believe that when we will the good of others and mimic the divine characteristics of God in our own lives, God becomes very present.

Hope, Thought, and Belief

Everything begins and ends in the brain *and* with our thoughts. I set out on a multiyear journey to improve my health and reduce my stress. Through my research and experience, I found that the traditional physical solutions didn't work by themselves. It was a nonphysical aspect of my life that was the key to improvement.

My goal was to achieve the greatest possible degree of health and well-being, which meant that I had to take my *thoughts* (and subsequent actions) to the highest possible level. Eventually, through that process, I achieved self-actualization—my fullest potential—in all areas of my life. I found that for me, self-actualization is rooted in the existence and nature of God. It is rooted in love, beauty, truth, goodness, free will, purpose, meaning, and hope. Not a naïve optimism or wishful-thinking kind of hope, but a conviction that good will ultimately prevail.

Bishop Robert Barron, auxiliary bishop of the archdiocese of Los Angeles and founder of the Word on Fire ministries, defines hope as "a trust in the ultimate sovereignty of God."[5] This means that in the end, because God is perfect love and goodness and in charge of all creation, all will be well. That may be hard to process, particularly in times of suffering, but it is not irrational.

The optimistic views of Leibniz and Craig are just two examples of ways in which I use my free will in thinking, based in logic and the notion of God, to cope with stress and difficulty. Thinking in the way of those philosophers gives me a profound sense of hope, which helps me relax in times of distress and muster a confident outlook. In addition to self-actualization and the numerous reasons I've described in this book, hope is *why* I choose God.

People who have a strong sense of hope or an optimistic outlook on life have stronger relationships and greater resilience, are more productive at work, and are happier than those who do not.[6] Not only does the notion of God bring love, goodness, beauty, and truth (all of which, as we know, have significant health benefits) into my life, but belief in the existence and nature of God provides an optimistic foundation for my worldview.

To feel that right now, in this very moment, the creator of the universe, the source and standard of love and goodness, is willing the good in my life, with every breath I take and every beat of my heart, is indescribable. We are always free to choose the way we view the world and process the events that occur around us. I choose to look at the world in a way that helps when doubts creep in about my purpose, my future, or God's existence.

When I consider the many logical arguments for God's existence, and that God's nature is that of perfect love and goodness, it gives me great hope that I can overcome the challenges that enter my own life, because I have attributes that mimic the divine. If God exists, life has an ultimate purpose and meaning, and having a purpose in life leads to greater health and fulfillment. When I put myself in the shoes of the creator and try to be perfect in every possible way (willing the good of others at all times, being empathetic in every situation, trying to make someone's day a little better with every interaction, going that extra mile), I feel the greatest degree of fulfillment.

Setting our minds on God—on perfect love, goodness, beauty, and truth—and trying to act in a virtuous manner at all times, under all circumstances—is what brings us the highest degree of health and well-being. God is the standard, the highest degree of living we can strive to attain. We shouldn't settle for being good. We should strive for perfection, because perfection exists.

Logic Mind & Health Wellness Index

The Logic Mind & Health (LM&H) Wellness Index is a self-assessment tool I created to track my progress in the five areas of life that have the most direct impact on my health and happiness: truth, love, relationships, purpose, and beauty. When I am functioning well in these five areas, my health and well-being are at their peak. I feel relaxed, happy, and empowered. So will you.

Because scoring is subjective and we can sometimes be unaware of our feelings, having an accountability partner can help you more accurately assess where you are on the index. The index is cumulative, meaning the categories build on one another.

The most important category is truth, which represents your beliefs, mindset, and outlook on life. It affects everything else in your life and is the foundation of the index. Start there. Next comes the ultimate purpose in life, which I've described as willing the good of others. Through honest communication and virtuous action, love builds connection. Strong and loving relationships give meaning to life and create a greater sense of purpose and fulfillment. Combine all these, and you can't help but reduce your stress, become a better person, and create a beautiful life for yourself.

Take this self-assessment twice: immediately after reading the book and after a month of consistent practice drawn from the actions described in Part 3. Circle the appropriate number under each category (1 = lowest value; 10 = highest value), add up your numbers, and multiply by two. This is your LM&H Wellness score. The best possible score is 100.

The goal is to raise your score between the first self-assessment and the second. In addition, ask a loved one, friend, mentor, or someone else close to you to complete an assessment of you and tell you their score. This will provide a sense of how others see you and where it differs from how you view yourself.

On a scale of 1 to 10, with 1 being completely imperfect and 10 being completely perfect, rate the following as it pertains to your life:

Truth - certainty with respect to your beliefs and worldview, hope for the future, confidence in your ability to change, outlook on life. (Opposites would include doubt and fear.)

1   2   3   4   5   6   7   8   9   10

Love - willing the good of others, general feelings of compassion and empathy, expressions of gratitude, quickness to forgive, virtuous action throughout the day. (Opposites would include selfishness, lack of compassion and forgiveness, mistreating others.)

1   2   3   4   5   6   7   8   9   10

Relationships - open and honest communication with your loved ones, friends, and colleagues, enjoyable experiences with them, willingness to put aside what you want for what others want or need. (Opposites would include being dishonest or untrustworthy, cold or selfish, toxic interactions with people closest to you.)

1   2   3   4   5   6   7   8   9   10

Purpose - fulfilling your life's work, personal growth, stepping outside of your comfort zone, doing what you love to do and when you want to do it, making significant contributions to the world. (Opposites would include stagnation, feeling stuck or bored, not contributing to something greater than yourself.)

1   2   3   4   5   6   7   8   9   10

Beauty - feeling awe, wonder, joy, appreciation for nature and human creativity, able to be present in the moment. (Opposites would include narrow vision, lack of attention to or appreciation for things outside yourself, particularly things that should bring you joy.)

1   2   3   4   5   6   7   8   9   10

SCORE: _____

Journal

On the next pages are some questions to prompt reflection and facilitate self-expression through writing. The health benefits of these activities have been demonstrated through scientific research and Cognitive Behavioral Therapy programs.

This journal template should get you started. There are 30 pages, each with a question designed to encourage deep thinking and spark your creativity. Fill out one page every day. Once you have filled all the pages, create a journal for the next 30 days and beyond and continue writing down your thoughts and feelings on a daily basis.

What are your thoughts on the source of reality and how it relates to your well-being? What do you believe best explains your existence? Why?

What do you think about most throughout the day? When you sit in silence and focus on your breathing, where does your mind go? Are your thoughts healthy and loving? If not, why not?

What makes you happy? Is your happiness short-term or lasting? Is there anything that would make you happier? What is it? What can you do to make it a long-term reality?

What are you most afraid of? Why? What are the chances this fear will become a reality? Do you have negative thoughts about yourself? Do you have fearful thoughts about your life? Are they based in reality? What can you do to change them?

Did you suffer any trauma or hardship growing up? Do you relive those painful memories often? If so, have you ever talked to anyone about it?

What causes you stress? How does it feel physically? What thoughts occur to you when you are stressed out? What coping mechanism does stress trigger? What conditions or behaviors have you observed that elevate your stress level? Can you link those conditions or behaviors to similar experiences that were stressful?

How often do you will the good of another? How often do you go out of your way to sacrifice something or give up something you want or need for the good of another?

How often do you put yourself in someone else's shoes? How often do you see the world from another person's point of view? How often do you forgive those who have wronged you? How does it make you feel when you forgive or are empathetic?

Have you donated to a charity or other good organization, volunteered, or served your community lately? How did that make you feel? How could you make that happen more often?

What emotions are you feeling right now, in this moment? Why? What are some of the negative emotions you have been feeling lately, and why? What are some of the positive emotions you have been feeling lately, and why? What is the source of these emotions?

What are your habitual feelings throughout the day? What actions do they lead to? What would you like your habitual feelings and actions to be? How can you create these feelings and actions?

What do you do when you are stressed out or feeling anxious or worried about something? Do you talk to someone? Do you act out in negative ways? Do you express your thoughts and feelings or bury them deep inside?

Who can you open up to? Who else can you say these things to? Who opens up to you? What do you say? What do they say? Who else would you like to open up to you in this way? How can you make that happen? Do you admit things to yourself and open up to yourself before you can open up to others?

Who do you love? Why? What can you do to deepen that love? What could that person or those people do to facilitate that? Who else would you like to love, or love on a deeper level? What can you do to make that happen? How can you increase the love you have for yourself?

Who makes you feel alive and full of passion? How and under what circumstances does that occur?

How often do you take trips with your loved ones or experience something new and exciting with them? Where would you like to go? What would you like to do? How can you make that happen?

What does your ideal relationship with your family, your friends, your significant other look like? What can you do to turn that ideal into reality?

What are the talents and abilities you have that best serve others? What new skills can you acquire to better serve your purpose? What can you do to eliminate any roadblocks? Who can you get to help you?

If you could do anything with your life, what would it be? Would it serve others? Are you doing that now? If not, why not? What can you do to make it a reality? Who in your life can help you achieve it?

Why are you here and what is your ultimate purpose?

Do you have a passionate urge to do something big—e.g., write a book, create a website, build a business? What does it look like? Who does it serve? What can you do to get started?

What do you like to do for fun? Does it involve exercise? Nature? Human interaction? Is it healthy? How often do you do it? What new activities would you like to try?

What do you do when you want to relax? How often do you do it or these things? Is it right before bedtime? At other times throughout the day? Does it work?

Do you manage your time well? Do you make time for yourself throughout the day? What could you do to better manage your time at home, at work, with your extended family, with your friends?

When was the last time you experienced awe and wonder? What was that experience like? What other experiences could make you feel that way? What can you do to create more wonder and awe in your life?

How present are you throughout the day? Does your mind wander often or are you able to focus on the task at hand? What helps you focus and keep your thoughts from wandering?

What in your life is beautiful? What do you do or produce that is beautiful? Why do you consider it beautiful? How can you generate more beauty in your life and in the lives of others?

Do you have a daily mantra? Can you think of one now, write it down, and commit to reading it daily? Why did you choose the particular words or phrases you used to create it?

What is your daily routine: morning, evening, and throughout the day?

What does your ideal day look like? How can you make it occur every day?

Source Notes

Part 1

1. Joe Dispenza, *Breaking the Habit of Being Yourself: How to Lose Your Mind and Create a New One*, Carlsbad: Hay House, 2015, p. 128.

2. "'3-Brains-in-One' Brain," *PsychEducation*, 2019, psycheducation.org/brain-tours/3-brains-in-one-brain/.

3. Selena Bartlett, PhD, *Smashing Mindset: Train Your Brain to Reboot, Recharge, Reinvent Your Life*, San Francisco: Thrive Publishing, 2017, p. 7.

4. Marianne Szegedy-Maszak, "Mysteries of the Mind: Your Unconscious Is Making Your Everyday Decisions," *U.S. News and World Report*, Feb. 28, 2005.

5. Bruce Lipton, *The Biology of Belief: Unleashing the Power of Consciousness, Matter and Miracles*, Carlsbad: Hay House, 2005, p. 98.

6. Frank G. Lawlis, *The Stress Answer: Train Your Brain to Conquer Depression and Anxiety in 45 Days*, New York: Penguin Group, 2009, pp. 149-152.

7. "Chronic Stress Puts Your Health at Risk," Mayo Clinic Healthy Lifestyle website, March 19, 2019, mayoclinic.org/healthy-lifestyle/stress-management/in-depth/stress/art-20046037.

8. Natalie Rahhal, "MIT Finds Stress Can Cause You to Make Risky Decisions," *DailyMail.com*, Nov. 16, 2017,

dailymail.co.uk/health/article-5089925/Make-wrong-career-Stress-blame.html.

9. Lawlis, *The Stress Answer*, p. 21.

10. Dispenza, *Breaking the Habit of Being Yourself*, pp. 191-193.

11. Rima Laibow, "Medical Applications of Neurofeedback," in *Introduction to Quantitative EEG and Neurofeedback*, by James Evans and Andrew Abarbane, San Diego: Academic Press, 1999.

12. Lipton, *The Biology of Belief*, pp.132-133.

13. John Arden, *Rewire Your Brain: Think Your Way to a Better Life*, Hoboken: John Wiley & Sons, 2010, p. 4.

14. Mae Van Rensburg, "A Child's Subconscious Mind: How Parents Can Hurt or Help Their Kids," *Medianet*, March 18, 2017, medianet.com.au/releases/128343/.

15. Nadine Burke Harris, M.D., *The Deepest Well: Healing the Long-Term Effects of Childhood Adversity*, New York: Houghton Mifflin Harcourt, 2018, pp. 57-94.

16. Jill Bolte Taylor, PhD, *My Stroke of Insight: A Brain Scientist's Personal Journey*, New York: Penguin Books, 2009, p. 146.

17. Bartlett, *Smashing Mindset*, p. 9.

18. A.E. Moyer, et al., "Stress-Induced Cortisol Response and Fat Distribution in Women," *Obesity Research*, U.S. National Library of Medicine, National Institutes of Health, May 1994, ncbi.nlm.nih.gov/pubmed/16353426.

19. Len Kravitz, et al., "Cortisol Connection: Tips on Managing Stress and Weight," University of New Mexico website, unm.edu/~lkravitz/Article folder/stresscortisol.html.

20. Catherine M. Pittman and Elizabeth M. Karle, *Rewire Your Anxious Brain: How to Use the Neuroscience of Fear to End Anxiety, Panic, and Worry*, Oakland: New Harbinger Publications, 2016, pp. 28-29.

21. Michael M. Merzenich, *Soft-Wired: How the New Science of Brain Plasticity Can Change Your Life*, San Francisco: Parnassus Publishing, 2013, pp. 40-59.

22. Dispenza, *Breaking the Habit of Being Yourself*, p. 45.

23. Alvaro Pascual-Leon, et al., "Modulation of Muscle Responses Evoked by Transcranial Magnetic Stimulation During the Acquisition of New Fine Motor Skills," *Journal of Neurophysiology,* vol. 74.3, 1995, pp. 1037-1045.

24. Carmine Gallo, "3 Daily Habits of Peak Performers, According to Michael Phelps' Coach," *Forbes*, Aug. 8, 2016, forbes.com/sites/carminegallo/2016/05/24/3-daily-habits-of-peak-performers-according-to-michael-phelps-coach/#2c69c4c102cc.

25. Caroline Leaf, PhD, *Switch on Your Brain: The Key to Peak Happiness, Thinking and Health*, Grand Rapids: Baker Books, 2015, pp. 175-176.

26. Gallo, "3 Daily Habits of Peak Performers, According to Michael Phelps' Coach."

27. J. Bruce Moseley, et al., "A Controlled Trial of Arthroscopic Surgery for Osteoarthritis of the Knee," *New England Journal of Medicine*, 347.2, 2002, pp. 81–88.

28. T.J. Kaptchuk, et al., "Placebos Without Deception: A Randomized Controlled Trial in Irritable Bowel Syndrome," *PLOS ONE*, 5.12, 2010, p. E15591.

29. Vrinda Varnekar, "The Thomas Theorem of Sociology Explained with Examples," *PsycholoGenie*, psychologenie.com/the-thomas-theorem-of-sociology-explained-with-examples.

30. Lissa Rankin, "Scientific Proof That Negative Beliefs Harm Your Health," *Mindbodygreen*, June 12, 2015, mindbodygreen.com/0-9690/scientific-proof-that-negative-beliefs-harm-your-health.html.

31. Daniel Goleman and Richard J. Davidson, *Altered Traits: Science Reveals How Meditation Changes Your Mind, Brain, and Body*, New York: Avery, an imprint of Penguin Random House, 2017, pp. 165-190.

32. Sue McGreevey, "Eight Weeks to a Better Brain," *Harvard Gazette*, January 21, 2011, news.harvard.edu/gazette/story/2011/01/eight-weeks-to-a-better-brain/.

33. Goleman and Davidson, *Altered Traits*, pp. 98-99.

34. "Respiratory Sinus Arrhythmia," *ScienceDirect*, from *Goldberger's Clinical Electrocardiography* (ninth edition), 2018, sciencedirect.com/topics/medicine-and-dentistry/respiratory-sinus-arrhythmia.

35. Ashley Miller, "Natural Ways to Increase Serotonin & Endorphins," *Healthy Living*, Nov. 21, 2017, healthyliving.azcentral.com/natural-ways-increase-serotonin-endorphins-8991.html.

36. Matthew MacKinnon, "The Science of Slow Deep Breathing," *Psychology Today*, Feb. 07, 2016, psychologytoday.com/us/blog/neuraptitude/201602/the-science-slow-deep-breathing.

Part 2

1. Belinda Luscombe, "Do We Need $75,000 a Year to Be Happy?" *Time*, Sept. 6, 2010, content.time.com/time/magazine/article/0,9171,2019628,00.html.

2. Carey Goldberg, "Materialism Is Bad for You, Studies Say," *New York Times*, Feb. 8, 2006, nytimes.com/2006/02/08/health/materialism-is-badfor-you-studies-say.html.

3. Robert J. Spitzer, PhD, "The Four Levels of Happiness," Spitzer Center for Visionary Leadership website, spitzercenter.org/what-we-do/educate/four-levels-of-happiness/.

4. "Aristotle Happiness Quotes & Sayings," *SearchQuotes*, searchquotes.com/Aristotle/Happiness/quotes/2/.

5. Spitzer, *Finding True Happiness: Satisfying Our Restless Hearts*, San Francisco: Ignatius Press, 2015, p. 68.

6. Neel Burton, M.D., "Man's Search for Meaning: Meaning as a Cure for Depression and Other Ills," *Psychology Today*,

May 24, 2012, updated June 21, 2019, psychologytoday.com/us/blog/hide-and-seek/201205/mans-search-meaning.

7. Viktor E. Frankl, *Man's Search for Meaning*, Boston: Beacon Press, 2006, p. 113.

8. Stephanie A. Hooker and Kevin S. Masters, "Purpose in Life Is Associated with Physical Activity Measured by Accelerometer," *SAGE Journals*, Aug. 7, 2014, journals.sagepub.com/doi/abs/10.1177/1359105314542822.

9. Romeo Vitelli, "How a Sense of Purpose Can Help You Live Longer," *Psychology Today*, July 6, 2015, psychologytoday.com/us/blog/media-spotlight/201507/how-sense-purpose-can-help-you-live-longer.

10. Mara Gordon, "What's Your Purpose? Finding a Sense of Meaning in Life Is Linked to Health," *Shots: Health News from NPR*, National Public Radio website, May 25, 2019, npr.org/sections/health-shots/2019/05/25/726695968/whats-your-purpose-finding-a-sense-of-meaning-in-life-is-linked-to-health.

11. Elizabeth Blackburn, PhD, et al., "Intensive Meditation Training, Immune Cell Telomerase Activity, and Psychological Mediators," *Psychoneuroendocrinology*, U.S. National Library of Medicine, June 2011, ncbi.nlm.nih.gov/pubmed/21035949.

12. James Hamblin, "Health Tip: Find Purpose in Life," *The Atlantic*, Nov. 5, 2014, theatlantic.com/health/archive/

2014/11/live-on-purpose/382252/.

13. Victor J. Strecher, *Life on Purpose: How Living for What Matters Most Changes Everything*, New York: HarperOne, 2016, pp. 12-13.

14. Jill Suttie, "Living with a Purpose Changes Everything," *Greater Good* magazine, Greater Good Science Center at UC Berkeley, May 20, 2016, greatergood.berkeley.edu/article/item/living_with_a_purpose_changes_everything.

15. Caroline Leaf, PhD, "We Are Designed for Deep Intellectual Thought—It Keeps Us Healthy!" *Dr. Leaf's Blog*, Drleaf.com, March 26, 2012, drleaf.com/blog/we-are-designed-for-deep-intellectual-thought-it-keeps-us-healthy/.

16. Katrina Walsemann, et al., "Effects of Timing and Level of Degree Attained on Depressive Symptoms and Self-Rated Health at Midlife," *American Journal of Public Health* 102.3, 2012, p. 557.

17. Christopher Bergland, "The Power of Awe: A Sense of Wonder Promotes Loving-Kindness," *Psychology Today*, May 20, 2015, psychologytoday.com/us/blog/the-athletes-way/201505/the-power-awe-sense-wonder-promotes-loving-kindness.

18. "Doing Good Does You Good," Mental Health Foundation website, Aug. 1, 2017, mentalhealth.org.uk/publications/doing-good-does-you-good.

19. Jamie Ducharme, "5 Ways Love Is Good for Your Mental and Physical Health," *Time*, Feb. 14, 2018,

time.com/5136409/health-benefits-love/.

20. Thomas Williams, "Saint Anselm," *Stanford Encyclopedia of Philosophy*, Stanford University, May 18, 2000, stanford. library.sydney.edu.au/archives/spr2013/entries/anselm/.

21. Frankl, *Man's Search for Meaning*, Forward.

22. Frankl, *Man's Search for Meaning*, p. 131.

23. Hara Marano, "Why We Love Bad News," *Psychology Today*, May 27, 2003, psychologytoday.com/us/articles/ 200305/why-we-love-bad-news.

24. Frankl, *Man's Search for Meaning*, p. 112.

25. Loren Toussaint, et al., "Effects of Lifetime Stress Exposure on Mental and Physical Health in Young Adulthood: How Stress Degrades and Forgiveness Protects Health," *SAGE Journals*, Aug. 19, 2014, journals.sagepub.com/doi/abs/ 10.1177/1359105314544132.

26. Alexandra Sifferlin, "Forgiveness Protects Against Stress and Mental Illness," *Time*, June 16, 2016, time.com/ 4370463/forgiveness-stress-health/.

27. Frankl, *Man's Search for Meaning*, p. 66.

28. Kathleen Davis, "Cognitive Behavioral Therapy: How Does CBT Work?" *Medical News Today*, Sept. 25, 2018, medicalnewstoday.com/articles/296579.php.

29. Alice G. Walton, "Research Again Finds That Talk Therapy Can Change the Brain," *Forbes*, Jan. 25, 2017, forbes.com/sites/alicegwalton/2017/01/25/research-again-finds-that-talk-therapy-can-change-the-brain/amp/.

30. Jonathan Moran, *Cognitive Behavioral Therapy and Dialectical Behavior Therapy for Anxiety: Everything You Should Know About Treating Depression, Worry, Panic, PTSD, Phobias and Other Anxiety Symptoms with CBT & DBT*, Weston: self-published, 2019, pp. 67-72.

31. Julianne Holt-Lunstad, et al., "Social Relationships and Mortality Risk: A Meta-Analytic Review," *PLOS Medicine*, Public Library of Science, July 27, 2010, ncbi.nlm.nih.gov/pmc/articles/PMC2910600/.

Part 3

1. Charles Duhigg, *The Power of Habit: Why We Do What We Do in Life and Business*, New York: Random House, 2014, pp. 3-19.

2. B.J. Fogg, PhD, "Forget Big Change, Start with a Tiny Habit," B.J. Fogg at TEDxFremont, YouTube, Dec. 5, 2012, youtube.com/watch?v=AdKUJxjn-R8.

3. Dispenza, *Breaking the Habit of Being Yourself*, pp. 204-207.

4. Hugo D. Critchley and Sarah N. Garfinkel, "Interoception and Emotion," *Current Opinion in Psychology*, vol. 17, Oct. 2017, pp. 7-14, sciencedirect.com/science/article/pii/S2352250X17300106. 5.

5. Tori Rodriguez, "Mind Your Body: Inward Bound," *Psychology Today*, March 19, 2015, psychologytoday.com/us/articles/201503/mind-your-body-inward-bound.

6. Richard M. Piech, et al., "People with Higher Interoceptive Sensitivity Are More Altruistic, but Improving Interoception Does Not Increase Altruism," *Scientific Reports*, Nov. 15, 2017, nature.com/articles/s41598-017-14318-8.

7. Gerald Epstein, M.D., and Barbara L. Federoff, editors, *The Encyclopedia of Mental Imagery: Colette Aboulker-Muscat's 2,100 Visualizations for Personal Development, Healing and Self-Knowledge*, New York: ACMI Press, 2012.

8. Christopher N. Cascio, et al., "Self-Affirmation Activates Brain Systems Associated with Self-Related Processing and Reward and Is Reinforced by Future Orientation," *Oxford University Press Academic*, Nov. 5, 2015, academic.oup.com/scan/article/11/4/621/2375054.

9. Dolores Albarracin and Sanda Dolcos, "The Inner Speech of Behavioral Regulation: Intentions and Task Performance Strengthen When You Talk to Yourself as a You," *European Journal of Social Psychology*, Wiley Online Library, June 23, 2014, onlinelibrary.wiley.com/doi/abs/10.1002/ ejsp.2048.

10. "Progressive Muscle Relaxation (PMR) Technique for Stress and Insomnia," *WebMD*, Jan. 20, 2018, webmd.com/sleep-disorders/muscle-relaxation-for-stress-insomnia.

11. Courtney Ackerman, "25 CBT Techniques and Worksheets for Cognitive Behavioral Therapy," Positive Psychology website, May 29, 2019, positivepsychologyprogram.com/

cbt-cognitive-behavioral-therapy-techniques-worksheets/
#cognitive-distortions.

12. Leaf, *Switch on Your Brain*, pp.181-185.

13. Susan Weinschenk, "When People Feel Connected They Work Harder," *Psychology Today*, April 22, 2016, psychologytoday.com/us/blog/brain-wise/201604/when-people-feel-connected-they-work-harder.

14. Arden, *Rewire Your Brain*, pp. 119-127.

Appendix

1. Edward Feser, PhD, *Five Proofs of the Existence of God*, San Francisco: Ignatius Press, 2017, pp. 9-15.

2. Anselm H. Amadio and Anthony J.P. Kenny, "Aristotle," *Encyclopædia Britannica*, June 28, 2019, britannica.com/biography/Aristotle/The-unmoved-mover.

3. "Best of All Possible Worlds," *Encyclopædia Britannica*, June 6, 2017, britannica.com/topic/best-of-all-possible-worlds.

4. William Lane Craig, "Moral Responsibility and Emotional Rejection of God," *The Good Book Blog*, Biola University Blogs, Nov. 6, 2015, biola.edu/blogs/good-book-blog/2015/moral-responsibility-and-emotional-rejection-of-god.

5. Bishop Robert Barron, "Bishop Barron on Faith, Hope, and Love," YouTube, Jan. 31, 2013, youtube.com/watch?v=PuyKsaj6GbM&t=18s.

6. Paula Davis-Laack, "Want Less Stress and More Happiness? Try Hope," *Psychology Today*, April 30, 2015, psychologytoday.com/us/blog/pressure-proof/201504/want-less-stress-and-more-happiness-try-hope.

Made in United States
Orlando, FL
26 July 2024